BREAST CANCER

RECOVERY MANUAL

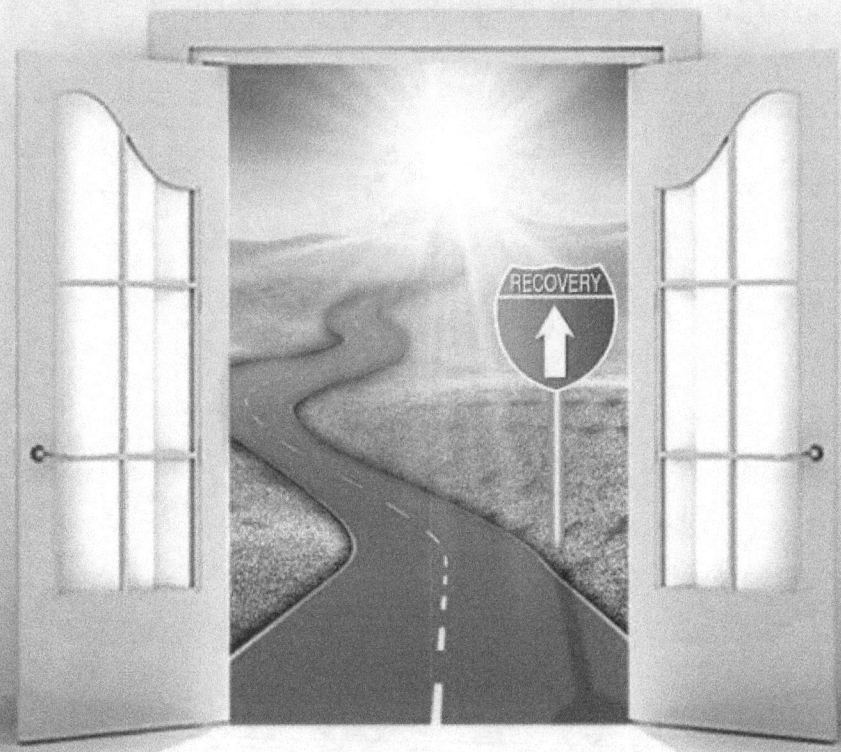

BY: EDNA CAMPBELL - MES, SURVIVOR

BREAST CANCER
RECOVERY
MANUAL

BY

EDNA CAMPBELL

SURVIVOR

FOREWORD

A few years after developing the Medical Exercise Specialist (MES) certification and workshop in 1992, we realized that MES was the first step in the new arena we had tagged as Medical Exercise Services. Since 1992 our Medical Exercise Specialists have encountered more types of clients in fitness settings than we ever expected.

A significant percentage of these unexpected clients are breast cancer survivors. Luckily the MES program has served as a catalyst for many of our graduates to use their experiences utilizing exercise as the primary modality in managing medical conditions they have personally encountered.

I have said many times, "Exercise is the key to long-term management of most medical conditions". Breast cancer is one of the conditions that certainly responds well to exercise. Breast cancer survivors demonstrate significant improvement in function, strength and range of motion, as well as reduced pain when engaging in an exercise program. But there was one missing piece...someone to step forward with the personal experience of living with breast cancer and the understanding of medical exercise sciences to develop a comprehensive exercise management process.

Then the catalyst stepped in.....my friend and colleague Edna Campbell. She has put together this fantastic manual based on her personal experience with breast cancer. This manual provides guidelines, exercises and tips to help breast cancer survivors use exercise to restore their function, regain their lives and help other survivors thrive and live a full life. Breast cancer is a condition that utilizes every aspect of medicine from the oncologist to the physical therapist to progress the patient to full recovery. Edna has now added the Medical Exercise Specialist to the list of professionals that progress the breast cancer survivor to full recovery.

The information in this manual is invaluable in giving breast cancer survivors a comprehensive exercise management plan.

Edna has broken down the exercise process into simple to follow steps breast cancer survivors at any stage can use.

Edna, thanks for being catalyst and sharing your wisdom, knowledge and courage to help others thrive and live.

Michael K. Jones, PhD, PT
1-888-610-0923
www.PostRehab.com

TABLE OF CONTENTS

INTRODUCTION

One day your life changed. You became a breast cancer patient, and then a survivor. I commend you for your resilience, and your courage to confront your battle and wake up every day to be a shinning ray of strength and hope for others.

If you are like I was, when you walked out of the cancer treatment center after your last treatment, or filled that last prescription for tamoxifen, you did not want anything to do with a cancer treatment center..........ever again!!!!

As you strode into the world of survivorship, inevitably, you recognized that although you have managed your diagnosis, you don't feel quite like you expected. Maybe you continue to feel fatigued or lethargic. Maybe bone pain is persistent, and maybe you continue to feel numbness and tingling in your extremities. All of this aside from the stiffness, and or swelling in your affected arm.

Yes, you have overcome, yet you still need some healing and strengthening.

The following pages will provide useful dietary, and exercise information to help you along your road to a complete recovery.

As this manual has been put together based on my personal experience, I encourage you to do your due diligence and further educate yourself on what is suggested here.

It is my wish that you become healthier and stronger than you have ever been. I encourage you to approach your recovery with as much fervor, focus and determination as you faced your treatment.

Yours in Survivorship,

Edna Campbell

Medical Exercise Specialist

For more resources to support your recovery please visit http://breasthealthrecover.com.

PROGRAM OBJECTIVES

1. TO EDUCATE ON THE IMPORTANCE OF DIET IN THE RECOVERY PROCESS.

2. TO ILLUSTRATE HEALTHY DIETARY SUGGESTIONS

3. TO INCREASE LUNG CAPACITY

4. TO BREAK UP YOUR SCAR TISSUE

5. TO IMPROVE MOBILITY

6. TO IMPROVE ALIGNMENT

7. TO IMPROVE MUSCULOSKELETAL STRENGTH

8. TO INCREASE AEROBIC ENDURANCE

9. TO REDUCE TENSION AND FATIGUE

10. TO PROMOTE A SENSE OF WELL-BEING

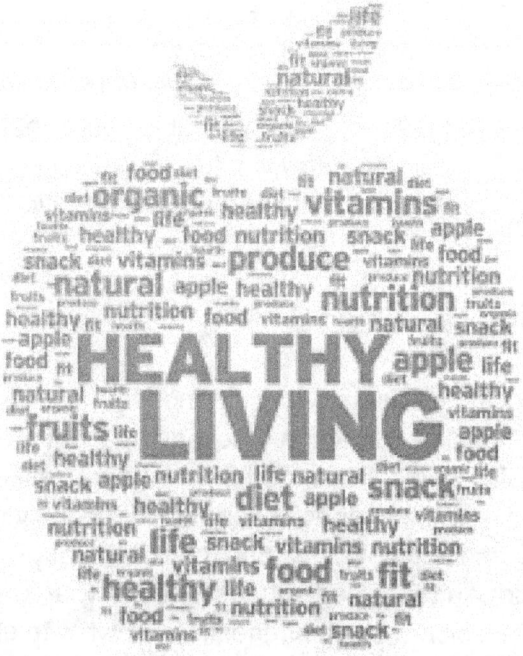

THE IMPORTANCE OF DIET IN RECOVERY

Your diet is the foundation of your recovery. In the process of ridding your body of cancer, your immune system has been suppressed, blood cell counts have been reduced, and all of your organ systems have been taxed. **Healthy cells have been damaged.** Now, you must focus on rebuilding and strengthening your body systems.

You cannot afford to not pay attention to your diet. According to the National Cancer Institute, malnutrition is the cause of death for approximately 40% of the fatalities of cancer patients, while nearly 80% percent of cancer patients become clinically malnutritioned. This often manifests itself in other weaknesses.

Proper nutrient and caloric intake should be of utmost importance as you recover and rebuild yourself. You must direct attention to how to nourish and fuel your body. What you put into your system will impact your energy levels, the elimination of toxic chemicals, and the regeneration and rebuilding of cells.

Request a copy of the results of your last blood work. As you peruse those results, you will probably notice that most of your levels are close to or below what is considered normal. Focus on getting those levels up. Time and proper nutrition will help.

DIETARY SUGGESTIONS

It should be understood, first and foremost, that that dietary and nutritional needs of the recovering patient are not addressed in the USDA's Recommended Daily Allowances. As we are recovering, we have special needs and probably need more nutrients and supplements than the RDA suggests.

In addition to making suggestions for what to add to your diet, we will also provide suggestions of what to eliminate. These suggestions are aimed at strengthening your immune system, building strength, and reducing your intake of toxins.

When we are educated and directed to properly nourish ourselves, it has been proven at Lifestyle Centers of America that it is possible to reduce the side-effects of treatment and create the landscape to live a life of vitality that is disease and ailment free. That is the purpose of the lists I have included below.

OVERALL GUIDELINES

1) Reduce/eliminate meat protein.
2) Reduce/eliminate dairy, especially cheese.
3) Try to use organic fruit and vegetables.
4) Eat more foods raw, rather than cooked.
5) Reduce/eliminate simple sugars.
6) Eliminate hydrogenated oils.
7) Reduce refined oils of all types. Replace with whole nuts and seeds.

To best support your program goals, consider these overall guidelines, and then try to select foods from the list of suggestions provided.

CARBOHYDRATES

Carbrohydrates are essential for brain function and energy. Replace refined "white" carbs with these whole food versions.
- Brown Rice
- Millet
- Organic Fruit
- Raw or Steamed Vegetables
- Whole Grains

PROTEINS

Reduce your intake of animal proteins and increase your use of plant-proteins.
- Tofu
- Lentils
- Beans
- Grilled Chicken
- Grilled Fish

FATS

You need some healthy fats in your diet. Use the whole seeds as often as you can and keep your use of the oils to a minimum. Make sure flax oil is refrigerated as flax oil oxidizes rapidly into a carcinogenic substance. This is not something you want to ingest into your system as you begin to maintain a clean body system.
- Olive oil
- Flax seed and flax seed oil
- Walnuts
- Chia seeds
- Coconut oil

DAIRY REPLACEMENTS

Dairy, even when organic, contains IGF-1, a hormone that has been statistically implicated in breast cancer risk. There are many nutritionally complete alternatives available today.

- Almond Milk
- Rice Milk
- Hemp Milk
- Cashew Milk

VITAMINS:

All of the following vitamins have been found to support recovery. The B vitamins are especially beneficial for calming the nerves so pain is more manageable.

- Vitamin A
- Vitamin B-6, B-12
- Vitamin C
- Vitamin D

MINERALS:

These minerals help your body's immune system and also improve pain management.

- Calcium
- Iron
- Magnesium
- Selenium
- Zinc

HERBAL /ALTERNATIVE SUPPLEMENTS:

Consider adding these supplements to your diet.

- Aloe Vera
- Beta 1,3 Glucan
- Green Tea
- Inositol
- Milk Thistle

FOOD PREPARATION CHECKLIST

1) Thoroughly wash and cleanse all produce, using the juice of one lemon to a sink half-full of water.
2) Boil, steam or bake. Do not fry.
3) Prepare food with stainless steel pots and utensils. Avoid aluminum.

RECIPES

PHYTO-BOOST SMOOTHIE

Ingredients

2 c. distilled water
8 oz. organic strawberries
4 oz. fresh raspberries
2 basil tops with the stem
1 1/2" sprig rosemary leaves
3 fresh mint tops w/stem
1" slice of ginger root
1/2 of a lime with the pith and seeds

Instructions

Place all the ingredients in the blender jar. Whiz together, on high, until smooth. ***Note:*** *If you want a frosty smoothie, you can freeze the berries and ginger root.*

GREEN MACHINE SMOOTHIE

Ingredients

3 c. distilled water
1/2 c. packed spinach leaves
1/2 organic cucumber
2 Swiss chard leaves
1/2 lime with pith and seeds
1 avocado w/seed
1 fist of parsley
1 small yellow beet
1 carrot
2 fresh basil tops/stems
1" slice of ginger root
1 Tbsp. agave nectar (optional)

Instructions

Place all the ingredients in the blender jar. Whiz together, on high, until smooth. **Note:** *Don't blend for too long as this oxidizes the nutrients.*

BROCCOLI BLISS SMOOTHIE

Ingredients

2 c. distilled water
1 broccoli stem (not the floweret)
3 Swiss chard leaves with stems
1/2 small red beet
1 ear of fresh corn cut from the cob
1/2 fuji apple with the seeds
1/2 lime with the seeds and pith
1/2 avocado with whole seed
1/2" slice fresh ginger root

Instructions

Place all the ingredients in the blender jar. Whiz together, on high, until smooth. **Note** _Don't blend for too long as this oxidizes the nutrients._

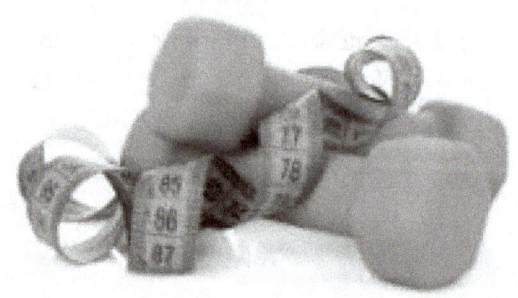

THE BENEFITS OF EXERCISE

1. Prevents health conditions and disease
2. Helps to manage weight
3. Improves moods(releases endorphins)
4. Increases Cardiovascular endurance
5. Improves musculoskeletal tone and strength

EXERCISE PROGRAM PRE~REQUISITES

1. Medical release to exercise
2. Completed all prescribed physical therapy and received a discharge.
3. No open wounds.

WARNINGS TO STOP EXERCISE

1. Chest Pain
2. Shortness of Breath
3. Any Numbness or Tingling
4. Light-headedness
5. Nausea

RECOVERY EXERCISE RECOMMENDATIONS

1. Wear loose fitting clothes, and shoes that provide traction and balance.
2. Read through and become familiar with each exercise before beginning.
3. Warm-up! Prepare your body for exercise.
4. Utilize proper exercise technique.
5. As you perform an exercise, focus on your body movement, and the purpose of the exercise
6. Exhale upon exertion for all exercises. Never hold your breath.
7. Drink plenty of water.
8. Cool down and stretch to reduce soreness, and prevent injuries.
9. Understand that healing and recovery are achieved over time, and we all progress at a different pace. Be patient and do not over-exert yourself.
10. Re-fuel within 30 minutes of exercising to optimize recovery.

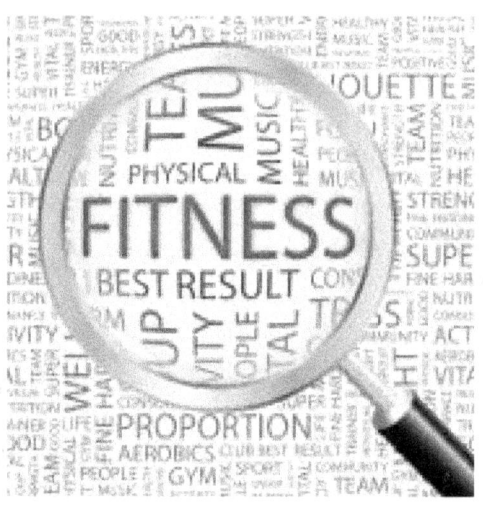

EXERCISE PROGRAM OUTLINE

As you scan the exercise program outline that follows, you will observe that we begin our path to fitness with a warm-up section. There's a very important reason for this. Warming up is very important for ensuring your exercise routine is injury free.

Warm-up exercises prepare your body for more vigorous strength-building activity. No matter what phase you advance to, you will never abandon the warm-up portion of your exercise routine.

The next phase in this exercise program focuses on improving your mobility. This includes focusing on core strength and functional strength, and increasing aerobic capacity. Aerobic exercise improves endurance, and the oxygenation of cells.

The last component of the program will provide you with some ideas and guidelines for ongoing personalized exercise planning. This will help to ensure your continued progress along your road to recovery.

WARM-UP

MOBILITY – PHASE 1

    a. Thoracic Mobility
    b. Muscle Recruitment
    c. ROM/Stretching

ALIGNMENT – PHASE 2

    a. Postural Training
    b. Balance
    c. Stabilization

STRENGTH – PHASE 3

    a. Core Strength
    b. Functional Strength
    c. Aerobic Endurance

PERSONALIZED EXERCISE – PHASE 4

    a. Personalized Strength and Conditioning

Now, that you have an idea of what's ahead on this recovery path, let's get started.

WARM~UP

Remember, no matter what phase you advance to, you will never abandon these warm-up exercises.

NECK STRETCHES

Ear to Shoulder Stretch

Exercise Check List
- Stand tall with head up. Look straight ahead.
- Keep your shoulders back

Exercise Instructions
- Bring your left ear to your left shoulder. Use your left hand to apply pressure and ensure a stretch. Hold for 15 seconds.
- Then move your Right Ear to your right shoulder using your right hand to apply pressure.

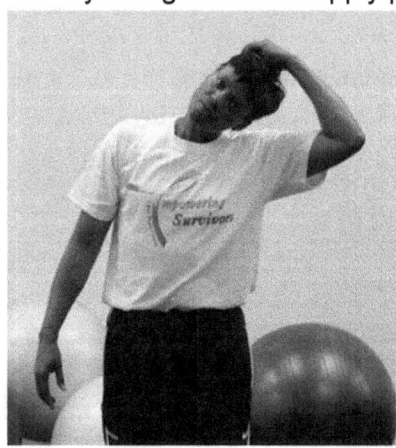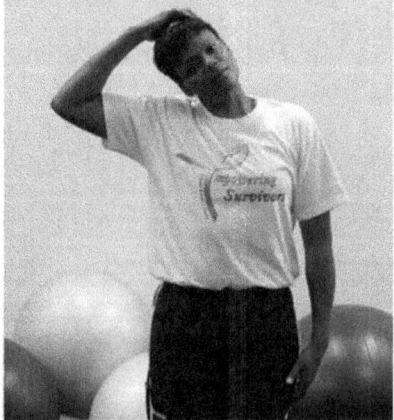

Progression as You Grow Stronger
4) Hold stretches for 15 seconds.
5) Work to where you can almost touch your shoulder.

Eyes to Ceiling and Chin to Chest

- Stand tall with head up. Look straight ahead.
- Keep your shoulders back

- Look up and slowly tilt your head back. Hold this stretch for 15 seconds.
- Then bring your head down slowly and touch your chin to your chest. Hold stretch for 15 seconds.

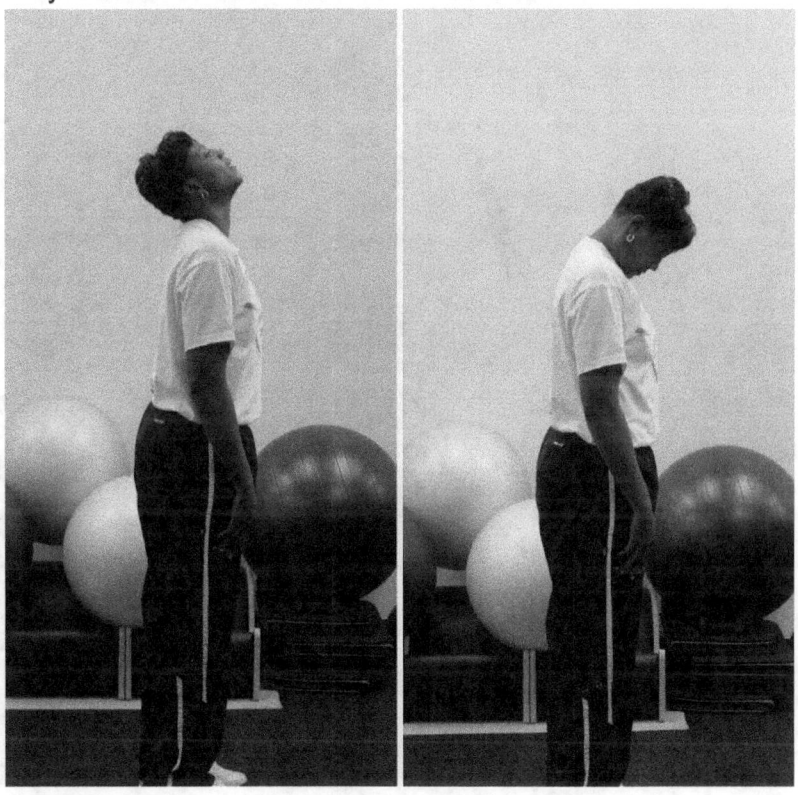

1) Hold stretch for 15 seconds on each side.

Neck Rotation: Right and Left

Exercise Check List
- Stand tall with head up. Look straight ahead.
- Keep your shoulders back.

Exercise Instructions
- Turn your head to the right and apply light pressure to ensure a stretch.
- Then, turn your head to the left and get the same stretch on the opposite side.

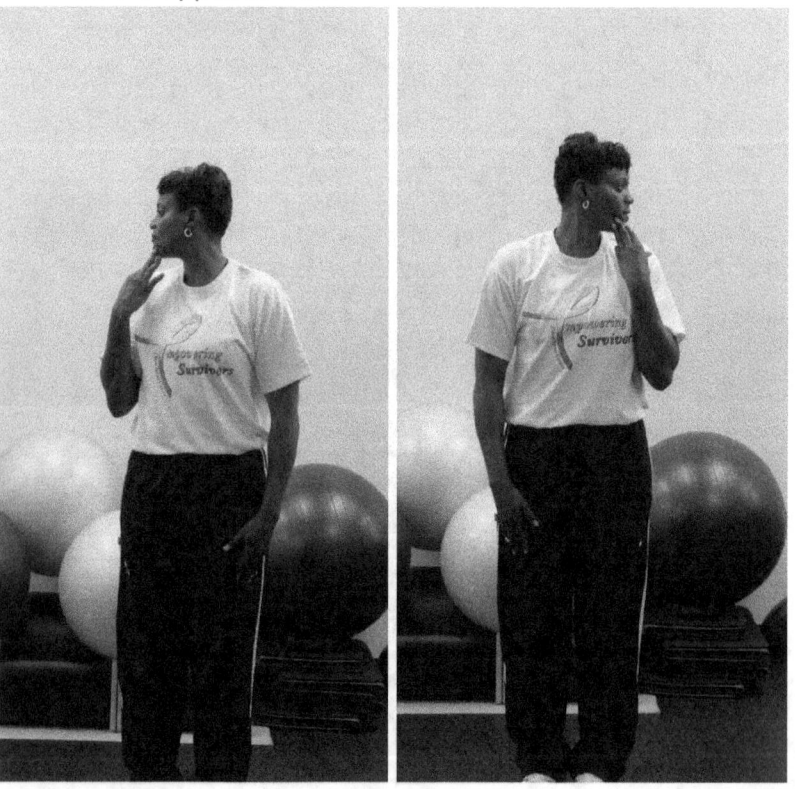

Progression as You Grow Stronger
1) Hold stretch for 15 seconds on each side.

Triceps Stretch

Exercise Check List

- Stand in a balanced and comfortable position.
- Keep your shoulders back
- Contract your stomach muscles.
- Place your feet shoulder's width apart.

Exercise Instructions

- Raise your right arm and reach for the ceiling.
- Bend your arm, bringing your hand behind you with your palm facing your back.
- Grasp your elbow with your left hand, and slowly pull your right elbow to the back.
- Pull the stretch as much as you can tolerate without pain!

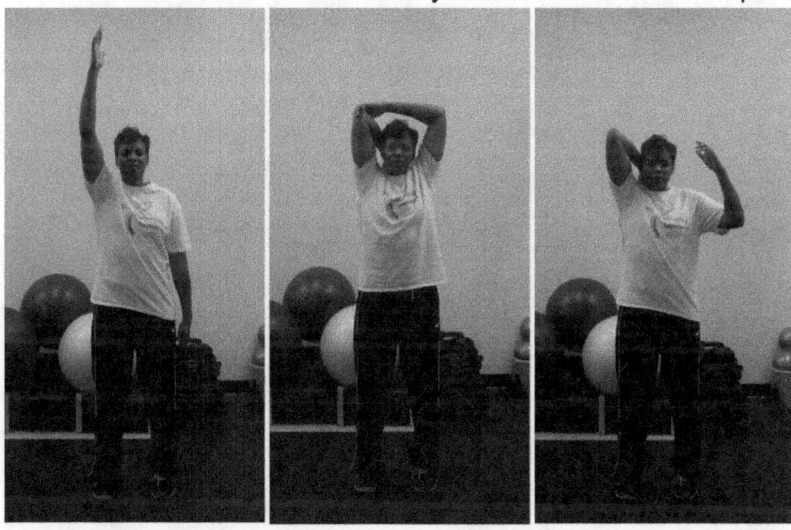

- Hold for 15 seconds.
- Switch arms. Perform the same stretch on the left arm.

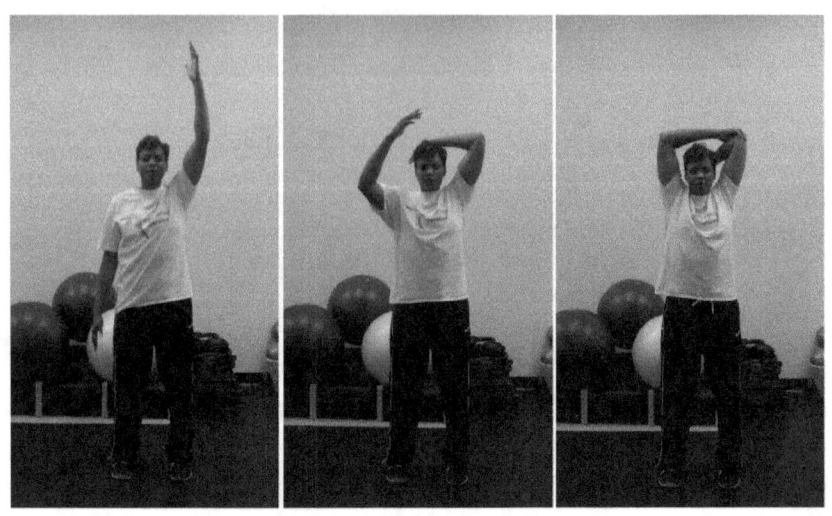

Progression as You Grow Stronger

1) Hold stretch for 15 seconds on each side.

SHOULDER STRETCHES

Arms Across Chest

Exercise Check List
- Stand tall with head up. Look straight ahead.
- Keep shoulders relaxed.
- Pull gently and stop if you feel any pain.

Exercise Instructions
- Lift your left arm and bring it across your upper chest at shoulder height.
- Keep your elbow straight as you pull your arm into your chest with your right hand.
- Switch arms.

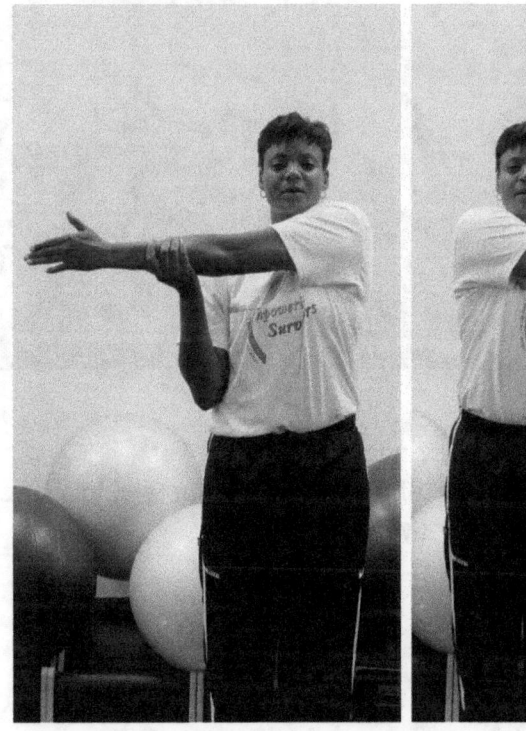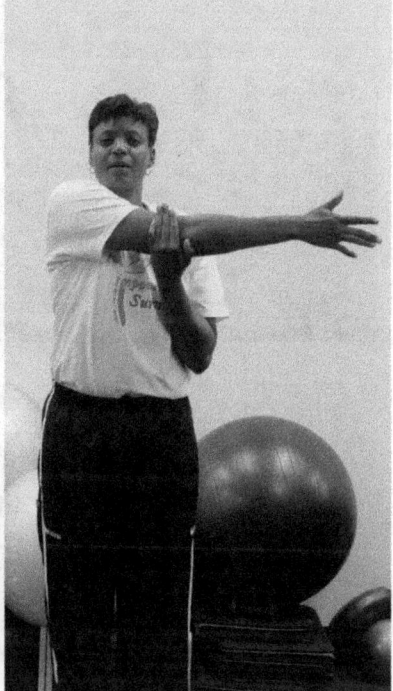

Progression as You Grow Stronger
1) Hold stretch for 15 seconds on each side.
2) Increase the depth of stretch gently.

LEG STRETCHES

Straddle - For Hamstring (Back of the Thigh) Flexibility

Exercise Check List
- Stand with legs straddled slightly wider than shoulder width apart.
- Focus on bending at hips, keeping back straight.

Exercise Instructions
- Bend down and reach for your toes on your right foot
- Gently move to center and place both hands as close to the ground as you can.
- Gently move to your left food and reach for your toes.

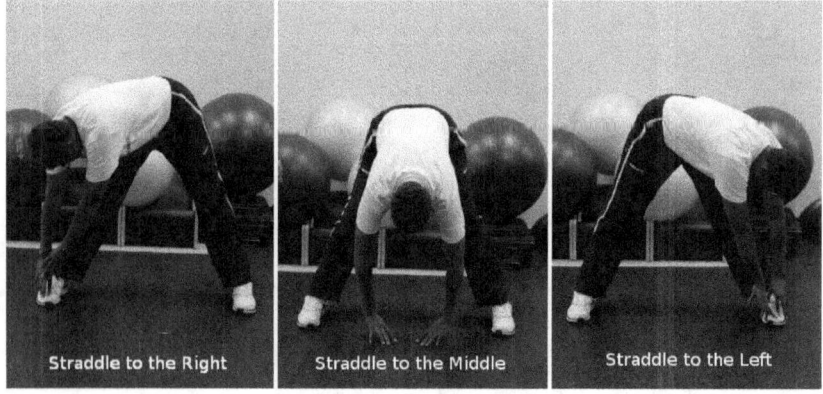

Straddle to the Right | Straddle to the Middle | Straddle to the Left

Progression as You Grow Stronger
1) Hold stretch in position for 15 seconds.
2) Increase depth of stretch until you are able to touch your feet and the floor between your feet.

Lying Quad Stretch - For Quadriceps (Thigh) Flexibility

- Lay down on your right side.
- Support your head and make sure your neck is not strained.
- Make sure your body is in a straight line.
- Keep your abs tight.

Exercise Instructions
- Bend your left leg so you can grab your foot with your left hand.
- Keep your knee in a straight line with your left hip.
- Pull back on your foot until you feel tension in your thigh.
- Remember to keep your knee level with your hip.

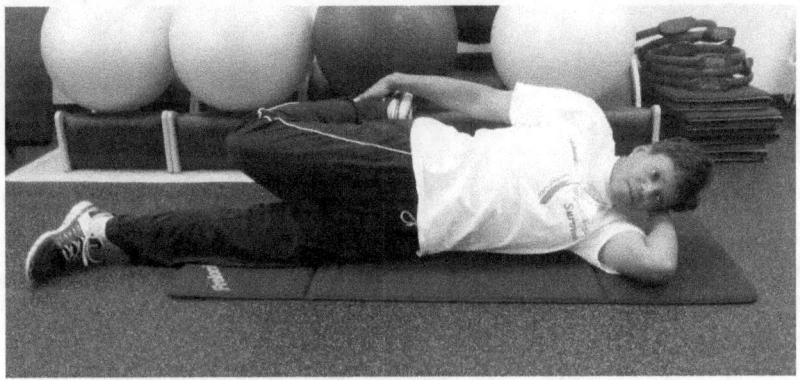

- Hold the stretch for 30 seconds.
- Roll to your left side.

- Repeat the stretch with your right leg.

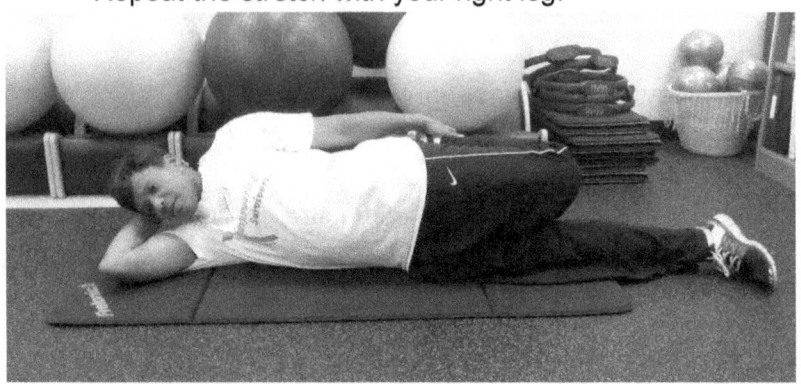

Progression as You Grow Stronger

1) Hold stretch for 30 seconds on each side.
2) Increase the depth of the stretch, but never stretch beyond what is comfortable.

Quad Stretch - For Quadriceps (Thigh) Flexibility

- Use a chair to maintain balance if necessary
- Stand tall with head up. Look straight ahead.
- Keep your shoulders back.

- Balance on your left leg.
- Pull the heel of your right leg toward your buttocks.
- Feel the stretch on the front side of your thigh.
- Switch legs.

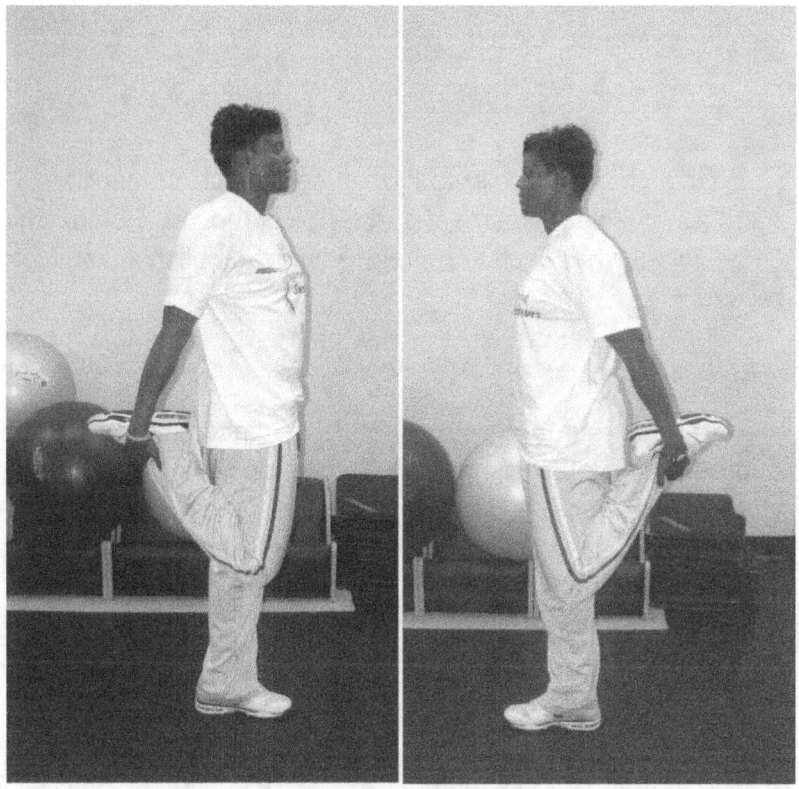

1) Hold each stretch for 15 seconds.
2) Pull the heel closer to the buttocks as it becomes more comfortable.

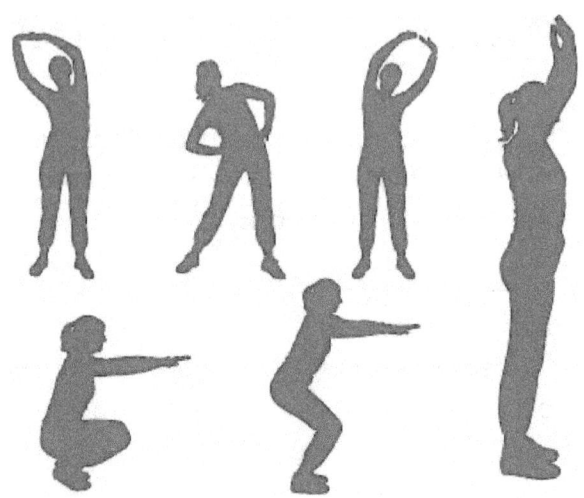

MOBILITY ~ PHASE 1

In this phase, we will work on three aspects of mobility—thoracic, muscle recruitment and range of motion/stretching. Let's look at what each area helps you accomplish in your recovery.

THORACIC MOBILITY:

After the trauma to your chest, it isn't uncommon to become guarded—to protect the area. You may tend to hold your arms close to your body, and not take deep breathes.

This protecting action is unconscious behavior, and it must be unlearned for maximum expansion of your rib cage and to increase your thoracic mobility.

Developing your thoracic mobility protects your spine from injury. The upper thoracic spine only flexes about 4 degrees between the T1 to T6 vertebrae. Your ribcage can to rotate up to a full 8 degrees across the entire T1 to T8 section of your spine. You can also strengthen your lateral flexion roughly 6 decrees between the T1 to T10 vertebrae.

The lower thoracic spine also benefits from exercise. Your bone structure may limit how flexible you can become, but achieving the maximum flexibility possible for both your upper chest and lower rib cage. The more flexible you are, the less likely you will be to have neck, shoulder, lower back and even leg pain.

MUSCLE RECRUITMENT:

This has probably not been the most active time of your life, and due to the inactivity, we want you to jump start your muscles back into action. We will re-teach your muscles to innervate, and feel comfortable contracting without going through each joint's full range of motion at this stage.

Start with the first level recommended. Confirm that you are able to handle it without excessive pain or discomfort. Resist the temptation to be discouraged by how "out of shape" you have become. Your muscles will respond quickly, especially if you don't overdo it.

RANGE OF MOTION/STRETCHING:

This component of the exercise program is meant to accomplish two things:
1) Break up scar tissue
2) Facilitate the activities of daily living such as putting on a shirt or putting groceries away.

Stretching complements muscle recruitment and thoracic mobility. It helps you get other areas of your body indirectly impacted by your surgery get into shape faster with a lower risk of injury.

MOBILITY EXERCISES

THORACIC MOBILITY EXERCISES:

Deep Breathing

Exercise Check List
- Head up. Looking straight ahead.
- Pull your shoulders back.
- Place hands on each side of your rib cage.

Exercise Instructions
- Inhale and exhale slowly (5 second count)
- As you inhale, you will feel your lungs expand and filling with air and your rib cage rise.

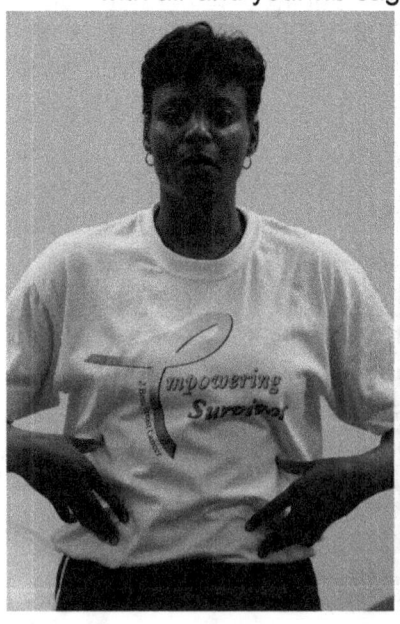 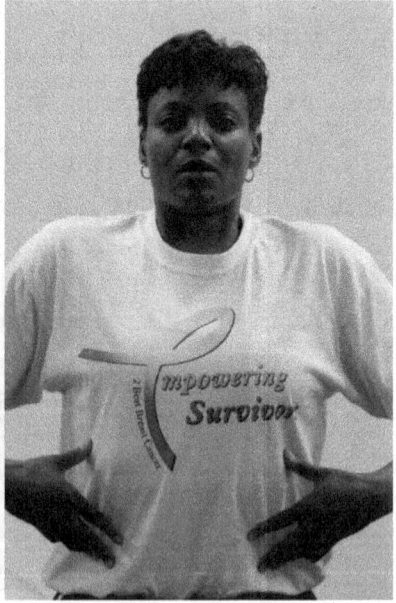

Progression as You Grow Stronger
3) 3 sets of 8-10 repetitions
4) 3 sets of 10-12 repetitions
5) 3 sets of 12-15 repetitions

The Wing Crunch

Exercise Check List

- Sit Balanced on a stool or physio (balance) ball.
- Keep your head raised.
- Contract your abdominal muscles.
- Keep your back straight.
- Keep your feet flat on the ground and do not twist your hips.

Exercise Instructions

- Clasp your hands behind your head as shown.

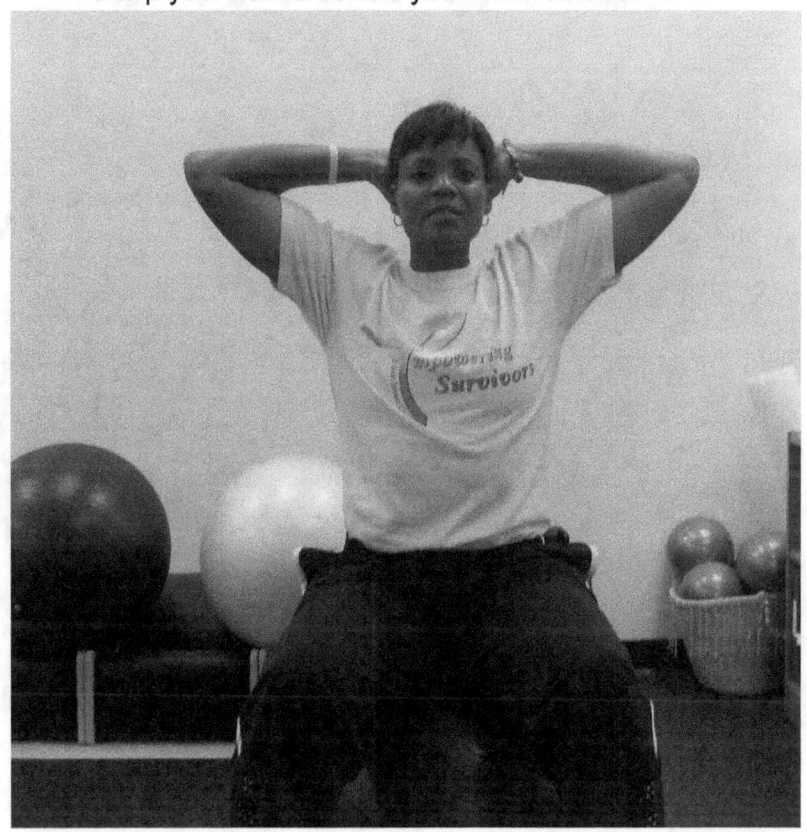

- Slowly turn your torso to your right. Remember to keep your feet flat on the ground and do not twist your hips.
- Turn to our right as far as you can comfortably turn without pain.

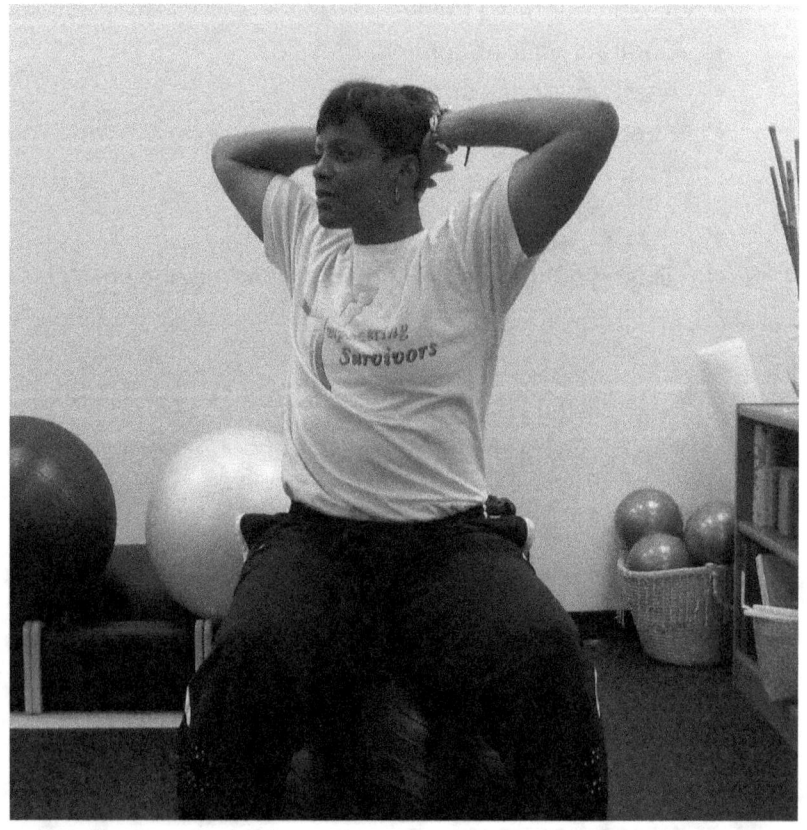

- Now, slowly lower your elbow toward the floor. This is the crunch.
- Exhale when crunching, or lowering your elbow to the ground.
- Return to starting position facing center.

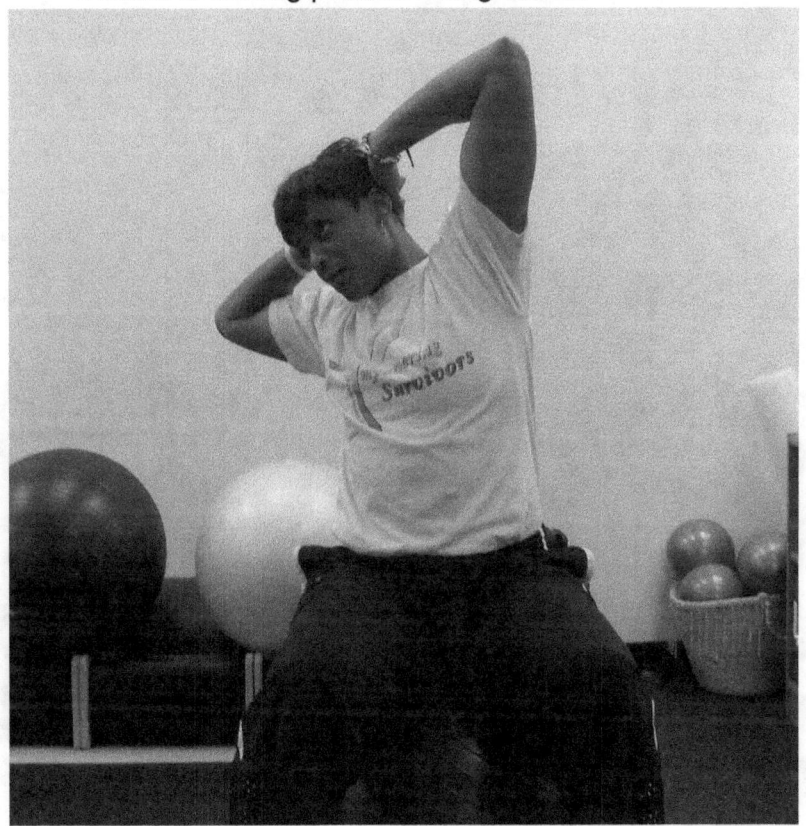

- Now, keeping your hips stable and your feet on the floor, turn to your left side.
- Turn your torso as far as you can to the left without pain.

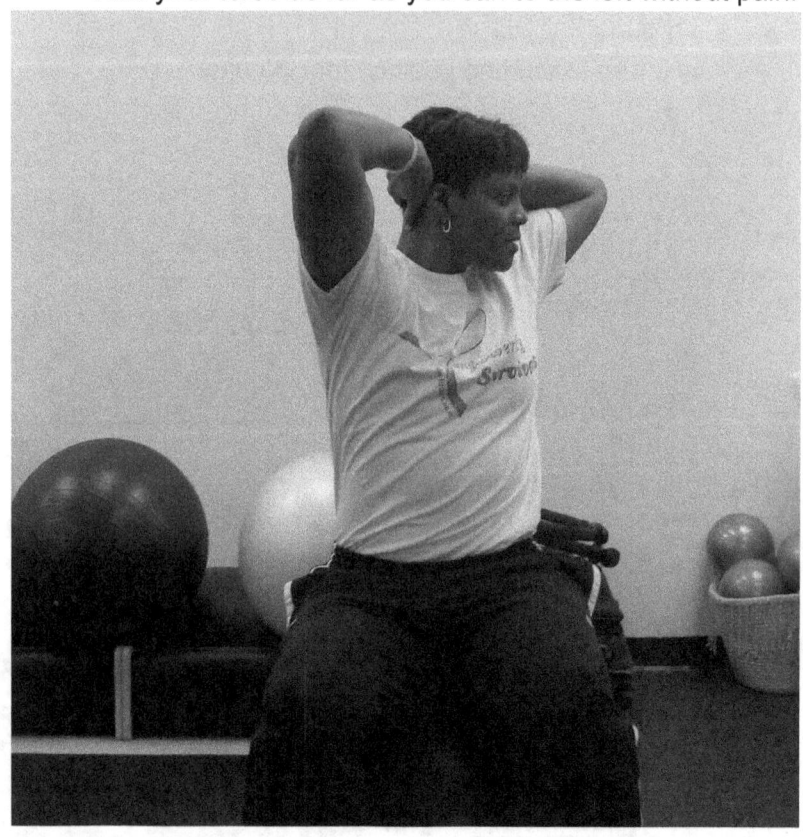

- Now, press your left elbow toward the floor.

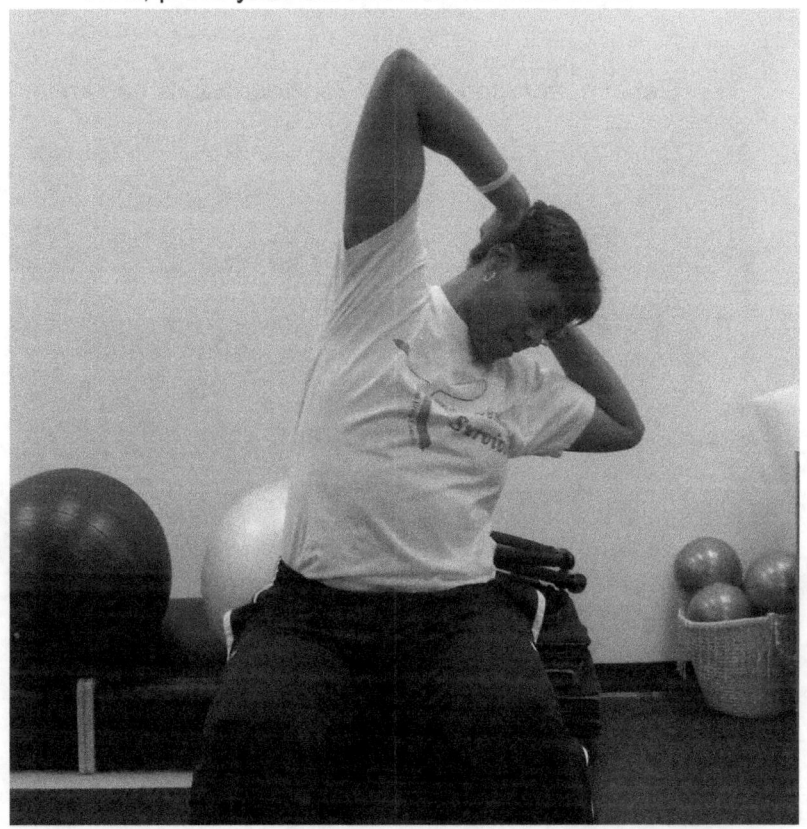

- Return to center before you begin the next repetition.

Progression as You Grow Stronger
1) 3 sets of 4-6 repetitions
2) 3 sets of 6-8 repetitions
3) 3 sets of 8-10 repetitions.

Wing to Knee

Exercise Check List

- Get in quadruped position (on your hands and knees).

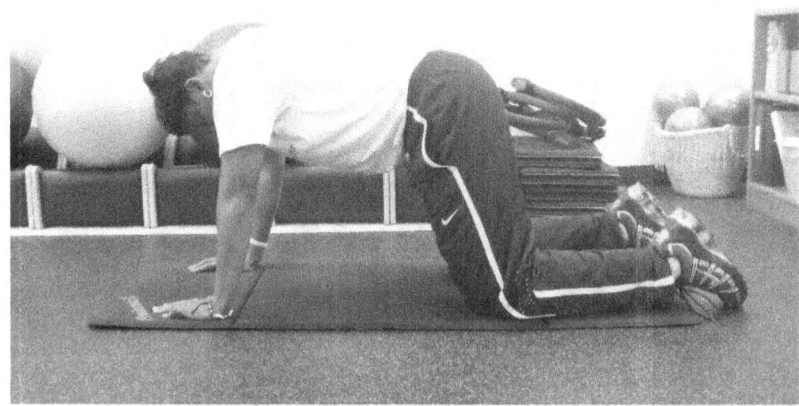

- Your head should be level with your tail bone
- Make sure your back is not arched.
- Keep your abdominal muscles tight.
- Keep your knees under your hips.
- Keep your wrists under your shoulder.

Exercise Instructions

- Place your left hand behind your head.
- Remain balanced on your knees, and do not twist your hips.

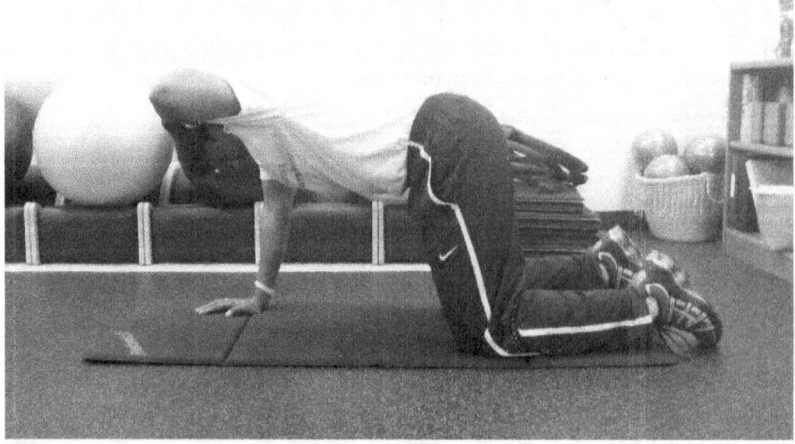

- Slowly, lower your left elbow to your right knee.

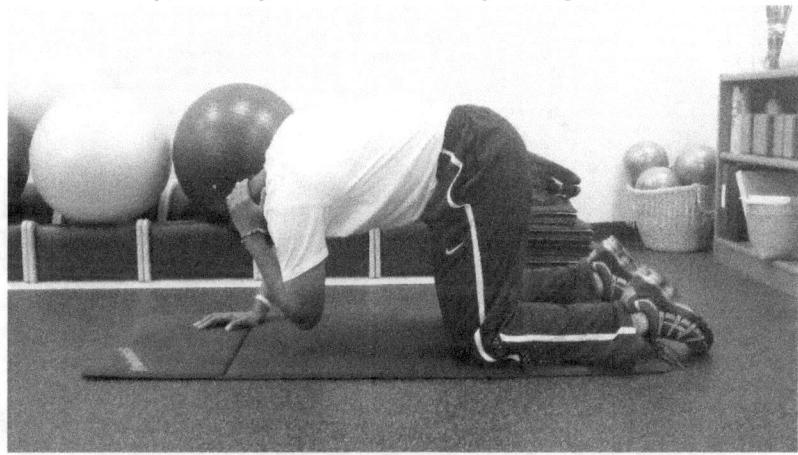

- Exhale as you lower your elbow.
- Keep your knees in place.
- Do not twist your hips.

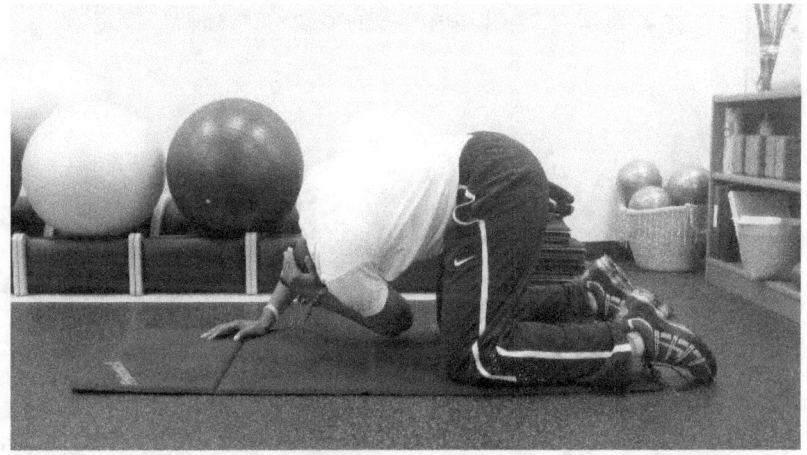

- You are striving to touch your left elbow to your right knee.

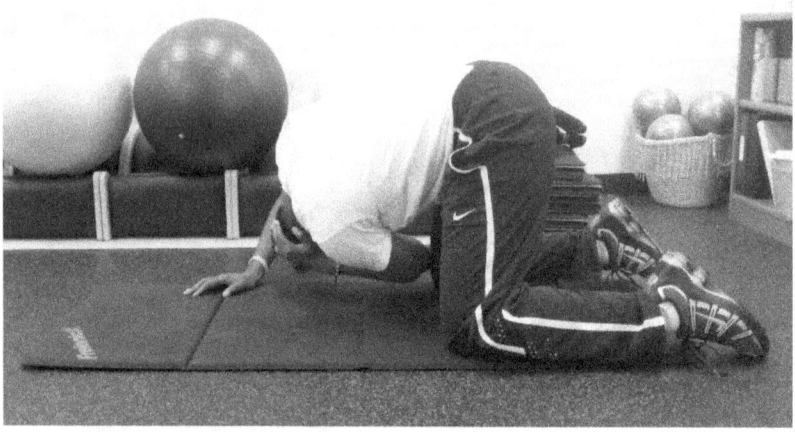

- Return to center position. Place your left hand on the floor.
- Place your right hand behind your head.

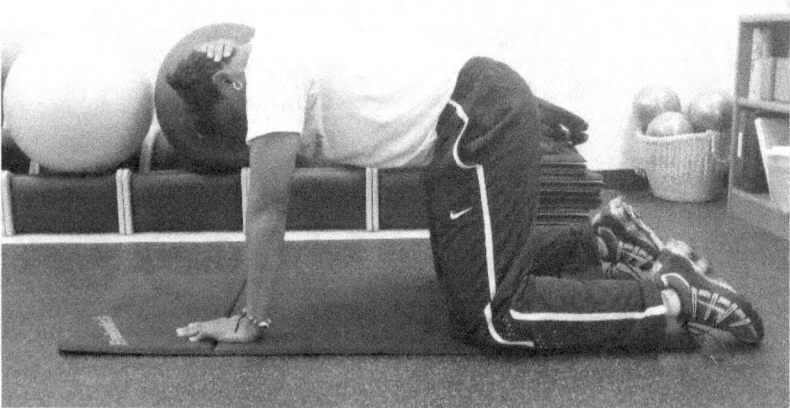

- As you reach your right elbow toward your left knee, exhale.

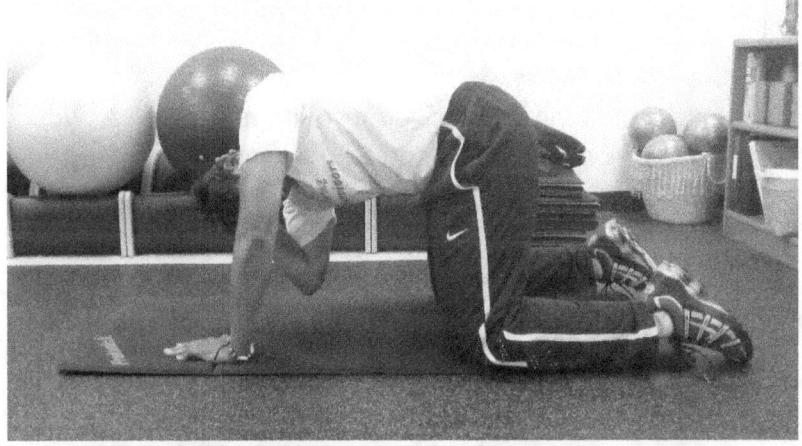

- Once again your goal is to touch the knee on the opposite side of your body.

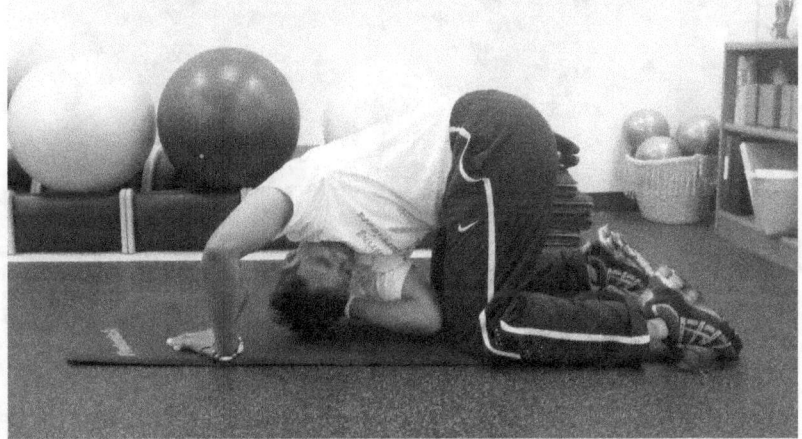

- Remember to keep your abs tight! And stop at the point you feel any pain.

Progression as You Grow Stronger
1) 2 sets of 6-8 repetitions.
2) 2 sets of 8-10 repetitions
3) 3 sets of 6-8 repetitions

MUSCLE RECRUITMENT

Hand Press

Exercise Check List
- Sit or stand depending on your fitness level. As you develop strength, sit on a balance ball.
- Keep your head up.
- Contract your abdomen.

Exercise Instructions
- Bring your hands together, locking the heel of one hand into the palm of the opposite hand.
- Press through each palm, creating static resistance.

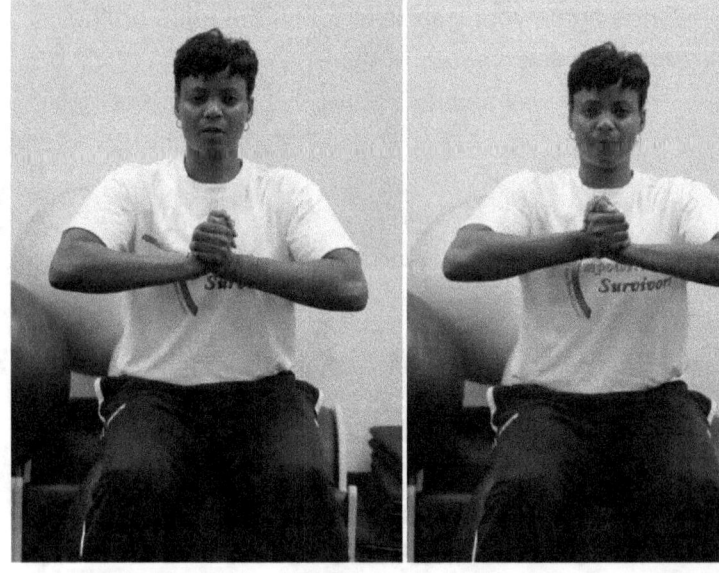

- Switch hands. If the fingers on your right hand were further away from your body to begin with, now the fingers on your left hand should be further away.
- You should feel it in your chest, triceps and shoulders.

Progression as You Grow Stronger
1) 3 sets of 8-10 second exertions
2) 3 sets of 10-12 second exertions
3) 3 sets of 12-15 second exertions

36

Elbow Tug

- Sit or stand depending on your fitness level. As you develop strength, sit on a balance ball.
- Keep your head up.
- Contract your abdomen.

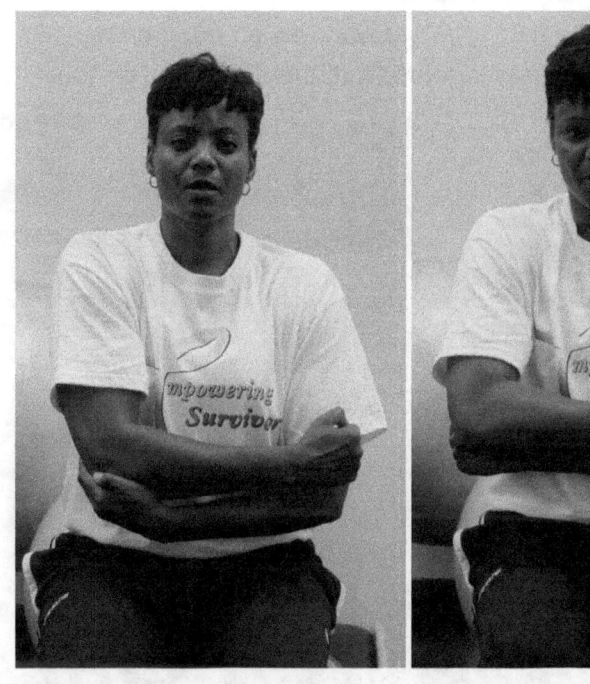

1) 3 sets of 8-10second exertions
2) 3 sets of 10-12 second exertions
3) 3 sets of 12-15 second exertions

Fist Pound

- Sit or stand depending on your fitness level. As you develop strength, sit on a balance ball.
- Keep your head up.
- Contract your abdomen.
- Keep arms at chest level.

Exercise Instructions
- Make a fist with both hands.
- Pound the fists together with the left hand on top.
- Pound the fists together with the right hand on top

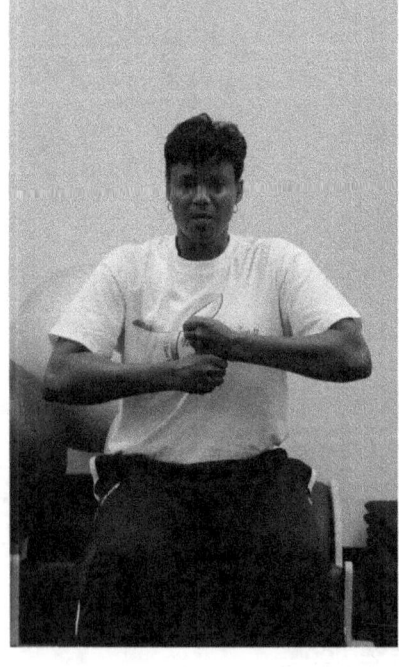 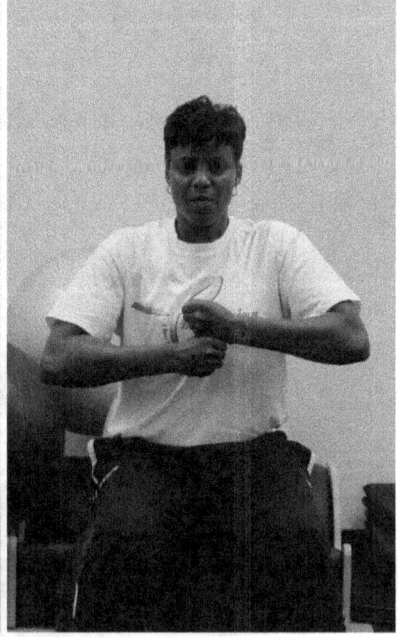

Progression as You Grow Stronger
1) 3 sets of 8-10 second extensions
2) 3 sets of 10-12 second exertions
3) 3 sets of 12-15 second exertions

Wall Sit

Exercise Check List
- Keep your back against the wall throughout the exercise.
- Press your back into the wall. Don't arch your lower back.
- Hold your abs tight.

Exercise Instructions
- Stand with your back to a wall, with your heels touching the wall.
- Keeping your back against the wall, bend your knees and walk your feet forward until your legs form a 90 degree angle.
- Holding this position for the time recommended for your fitness level. You will feel your quadriceps contracting.

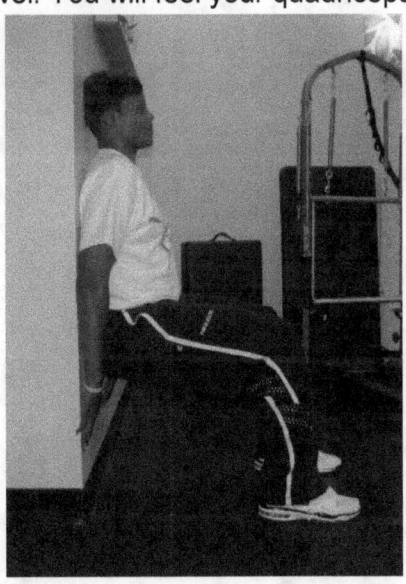

Progression as You Grow Stronger
1) 3 sets of 10 second holds
2) 3 sets of 15 second holds
3) 3 sets of 25 second holds

RANGE OF MOTION

Shoulder Shrug

Exercise Check List
- Keep your head level.
- Pull your shoulders back.
- Keep your back straight.
- Hold your abs tight.
- Place your feet shoulder's width apart

Exercise Instructions
- Let your arms hang freely at both sides.
- Raise both shoulders as close to your ears as your pain level allows.

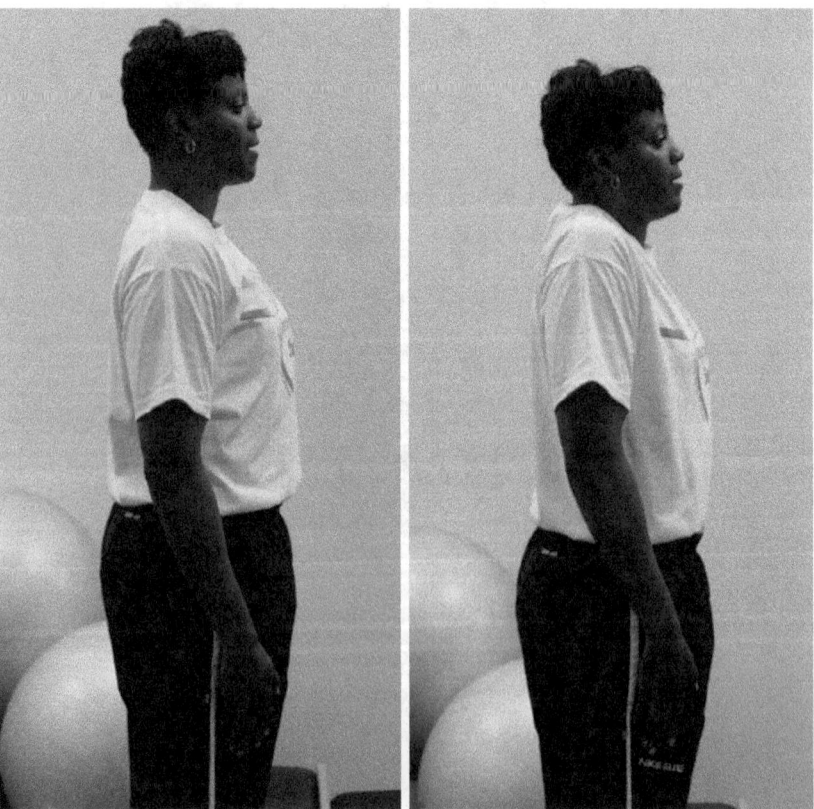

Progression as You Grow Stronger

Progression as You Grow Stronger
1) 3 sets of 6-8 repetitions
2) 3 sets of 8-10 repetitions
3) 3 sets of 10-12 repetitions

Lying Down Overhead Reach

The purpose of this exercise is to improve the range of motion in your shoulders. Your goal is to get to the point where you can place both of your arms flat on the ground above your heat. Don't expect to be able to do this early on. You'll achieve this goal gradually.

Our objective is for you to feel comfortable, knowing that this is a process. **You will experience progress over time. Don't get discouraged!**

Exercise Check List
- Lay down on your back with your knees bent to support your lower back.
- Focus your eyes on the ceiling.
- Keep your back pressed to the floor using your abdominal muscles. Don't allow your back to arch up.

Exercise Instructions
- Lay down on your back with your knees bent to support your lower back.
- Place your arms at your side with your elbows straight.
- Take a deep breath.

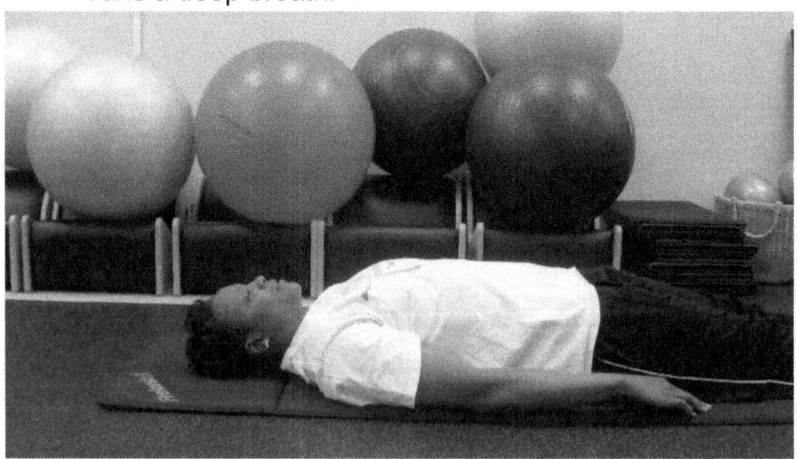

- Exhale slowly as you slowly raise both arms.

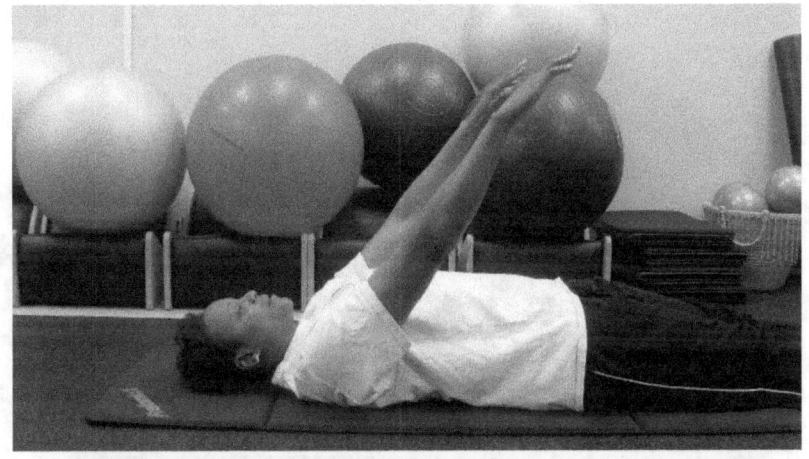

- Bring your arms up over your head as far as you can without pain.

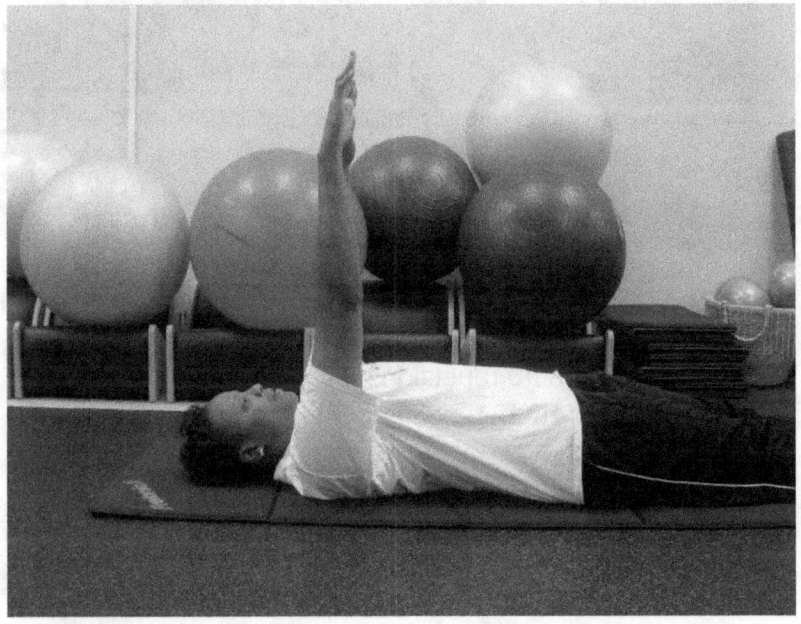

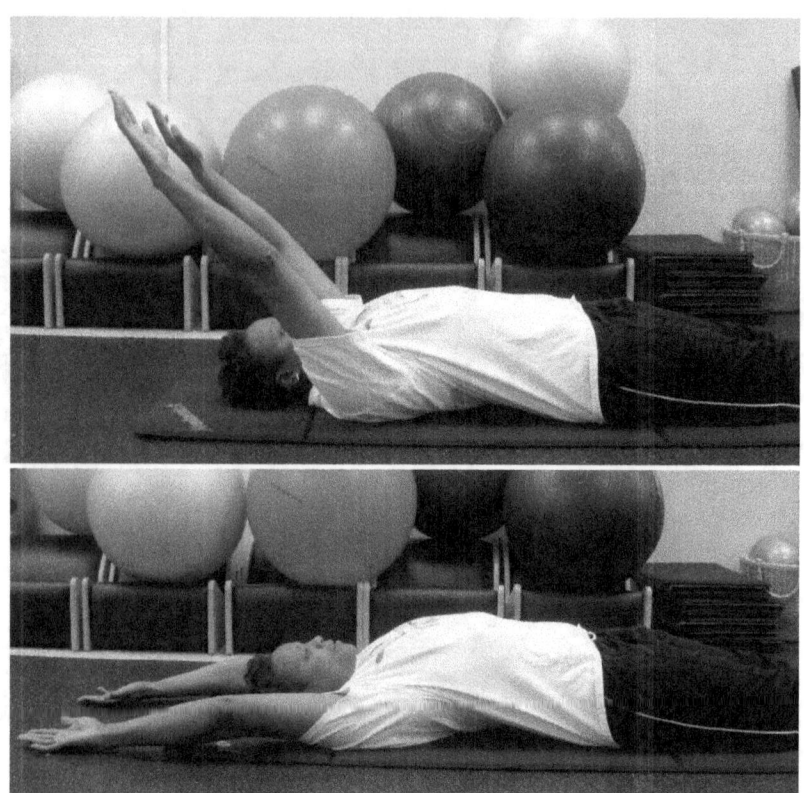

Progression as You Grow Stronger

1) 3 sets of 6-8 repetitions
2) 3 sets of 8-10 repetitions
3) 3 sets of 10-12 repetitions

Note:

You may alternate your arms if this is easier for you. Expect to feel some tightness in your chest and armpit when starting out. Be conscious, and know the difference between the tightness and pain. Pain is an indication that you have reached your limit and you should not be push beyond that range.

<u>*Front Raise*</u>

Exercise Check List

- Keep your head up.
- Keep your chin level to the floor
- Keep your back straight
- Tighten your abdominal muscles
- Find a dowel or piece of pipe.

Exercise Instructions

- Stand with your feet shoulder's width apart.
- Let your hands hang to your side.
- Grasp the dowel just outside your hips.

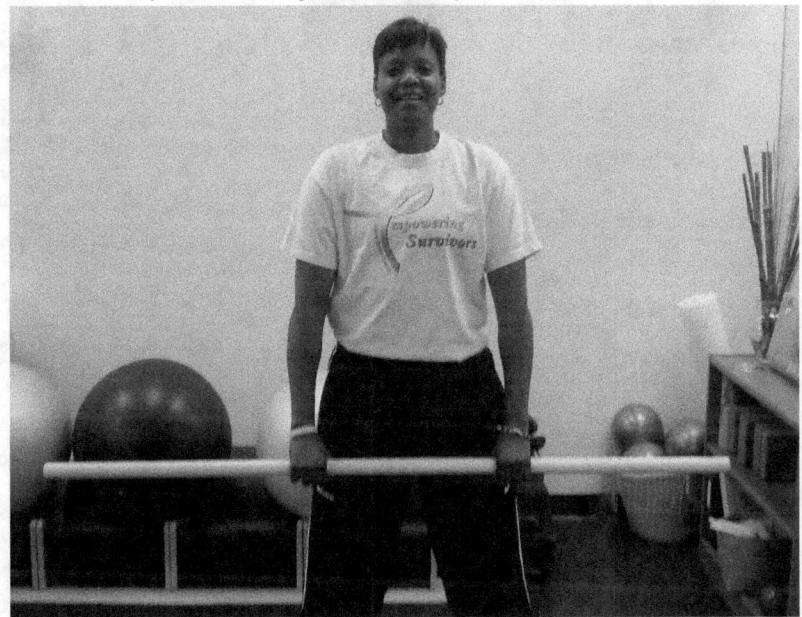

- Slowly raise the dowel in front of you.

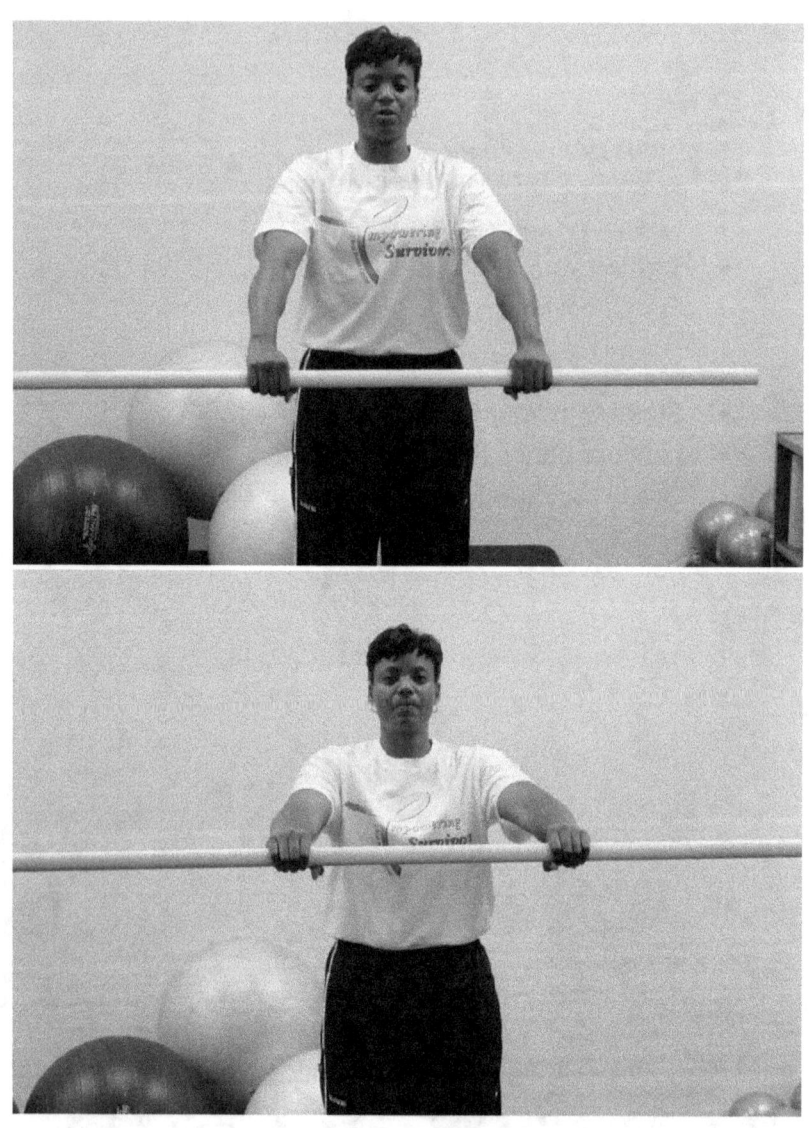

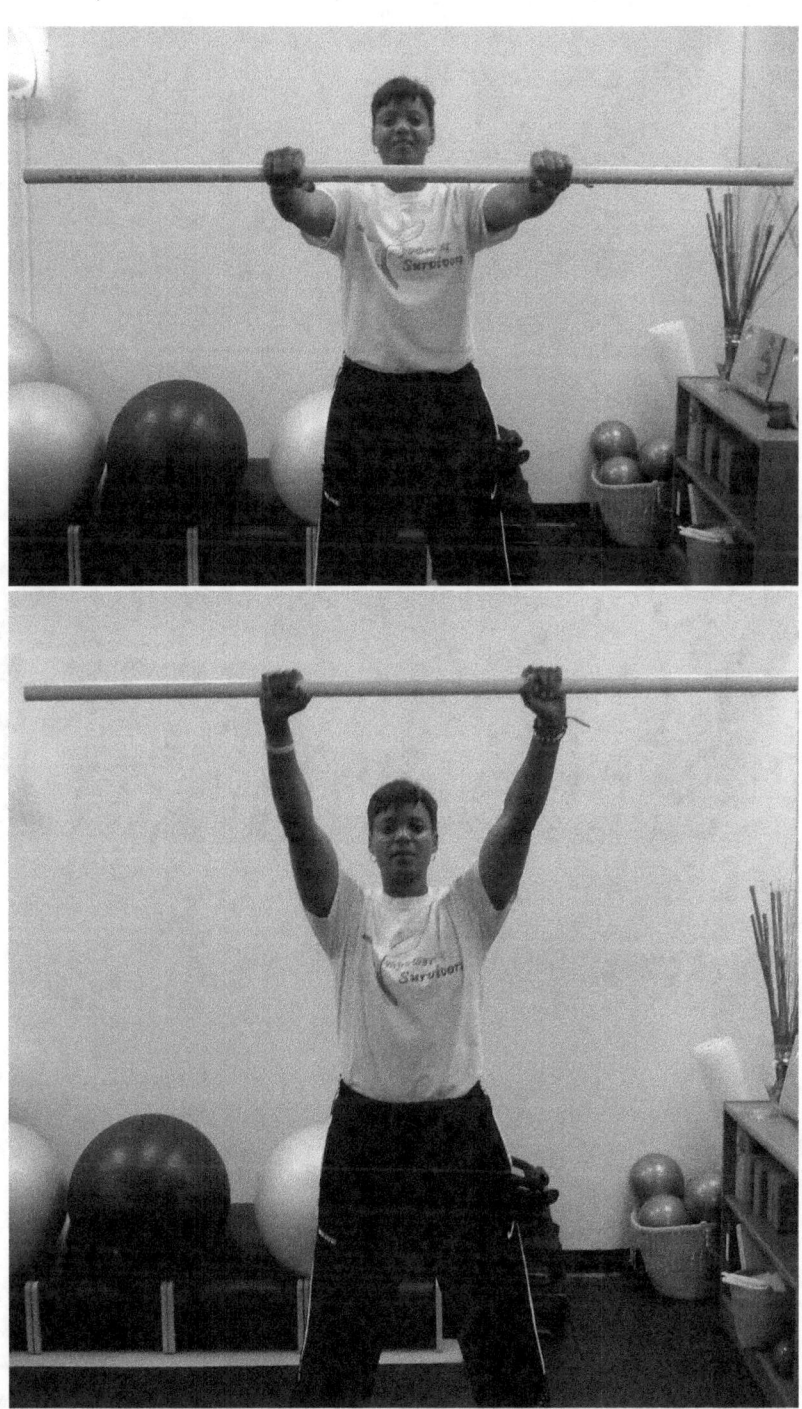

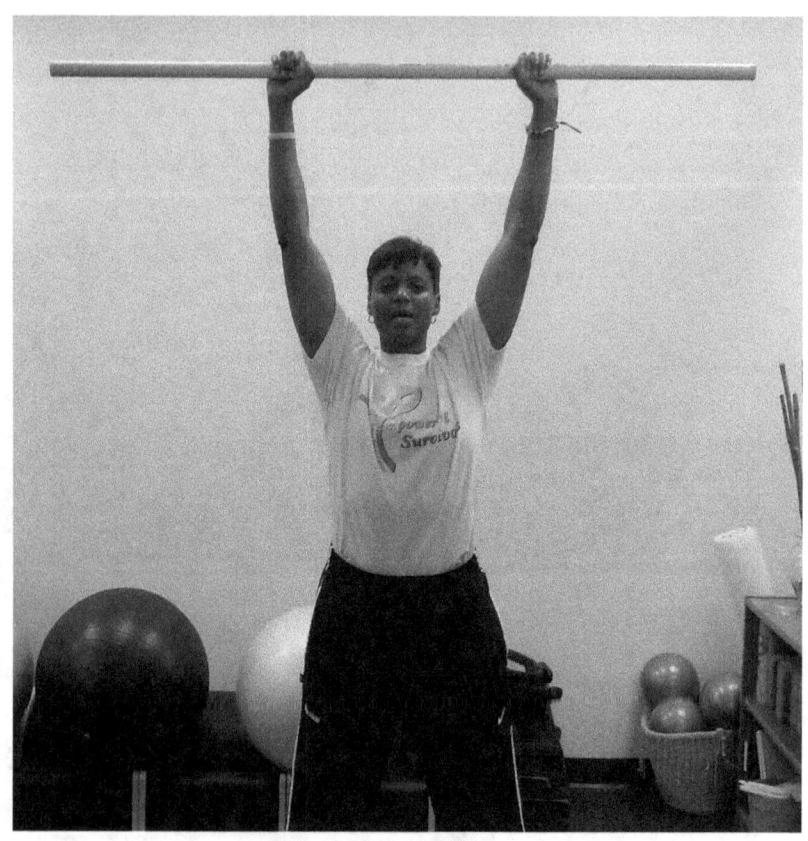

Progression as You Grow Stronger

1) 3 sets of 6-8 repetitions.
2) 3 sets of 8-10 repetition.
3) 3 sets of 10-12 repetitions.

Note:

You can also use a towel. If you do, pull your hands apart as you perform the exercise.

Rear Dowel Raises

- Keep your head up, your chin level to the floor.
- Keep your back straight.
- Stand with your feet shoulder's width apart.
- Let your hands hang to your side with your palms facing to the back.
- Grasp the dowel just outside and behind your hips.
- Tighten your abdominal muscles.

Exercise Instructions
- Slowly raise your arms behind you, keeping your elbows straight.

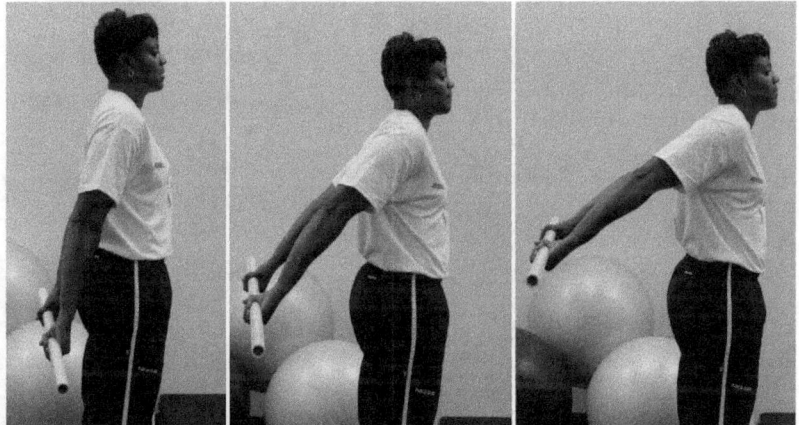

- Raise you arms only as high as you can without pain.

Progression as You Grow Stronger
1) 3 sets of 6-8 repetitions
2) 3 sets of 8-10 repetitions
3) 3 sets of 10-12 repetitions

Notes:

You may use a towel or exercise band for this exercise. If you do, pull your hands apart as you perform the exercise. This will activate more muscles.

Advance to more repetitions when the exercise ceases to be challenging. You can also increase the weight of the bar.

Front Wall Climbs

- Keep your head up.
- Keep your back straight.
- Place your feet shoulder's width apart.

Exercise Instructions
- Stand with the wall in front of you, with your toes touching the wall.
- Take one step back.
- Reach both of your hands towards the wall until your fingers touch.

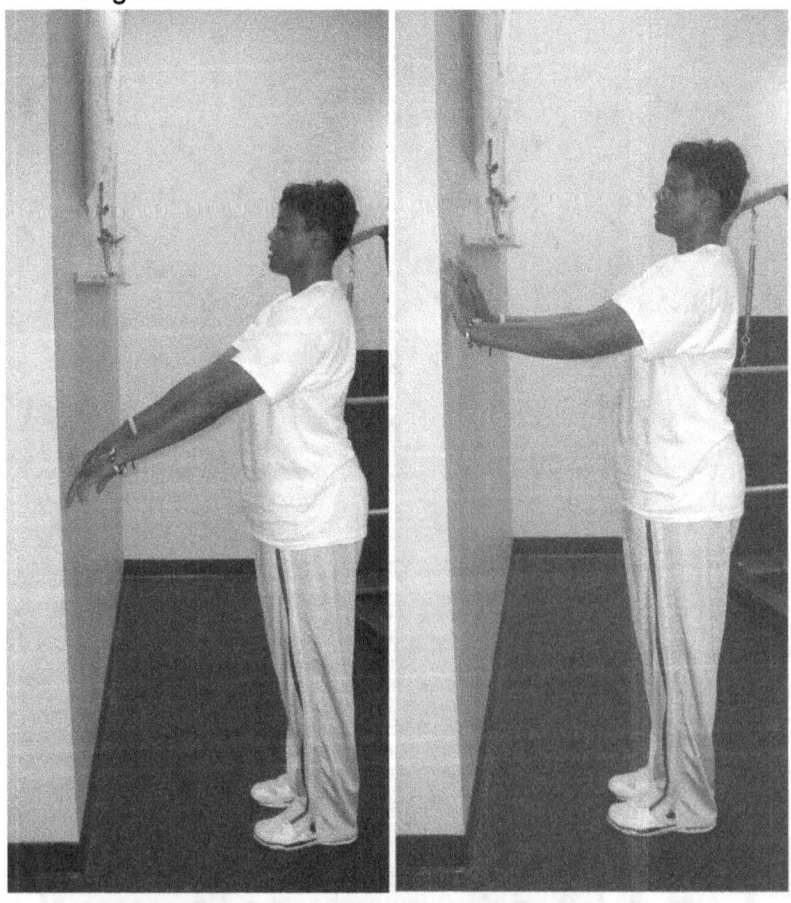

- Begin to climb the wall with your fingers.

50

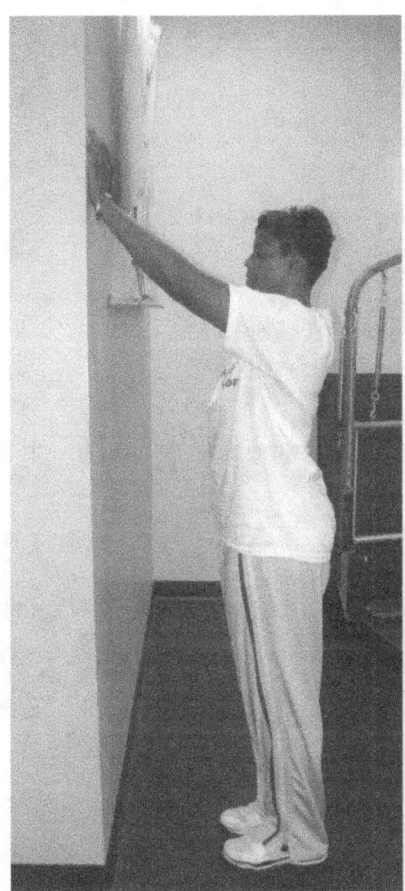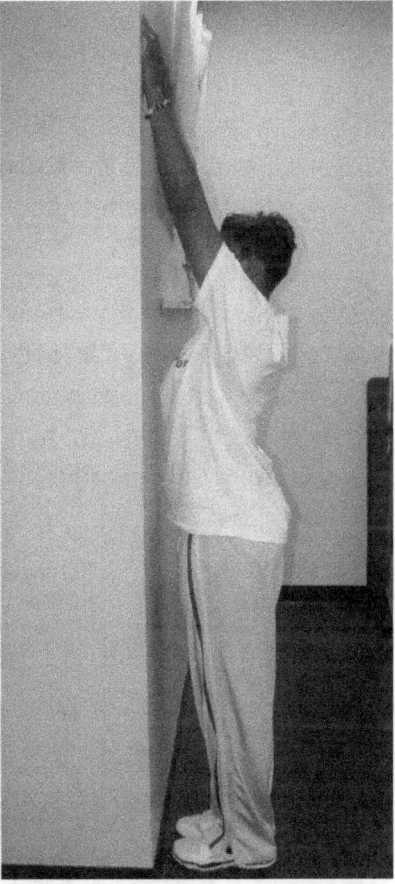

- As your arms gets higher, slowly step closer to the wall.
- Climb as high as you can without pain.

Progression as You Grow Stronger
1) 3 sets of 6-8 repetitions
2) 3 sets of 8-10 repetitions
3) 3 sets of 10-12 repetitions

Side Wall Climbs

Exercise Check List
- Keep your head up.
- Keep your back straight.
- Place your feet shoulder's width apart.

Exercise Instructions
- Stand with the wall on your right side.
- Begin with your foot close to the wall.
- Take one step to your left.
- Reach your right hand towards the wall so you touch it with your fingertips.

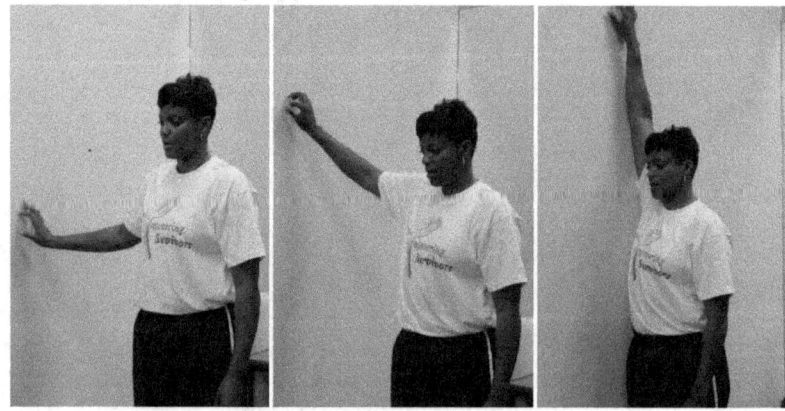

- Slowly begin to climb the wall with your fingers.
- As your arm gets higher, slowly step closer to the wall.
- Climb as high as you can without pain.
- Repeat on the other side as well.

Progression as You Grow Stronger
1) 3 sets of 6-8 repetitions
2) 3 sets of 8-10 repetitions
3) 3 sets of 10-12 repetitions

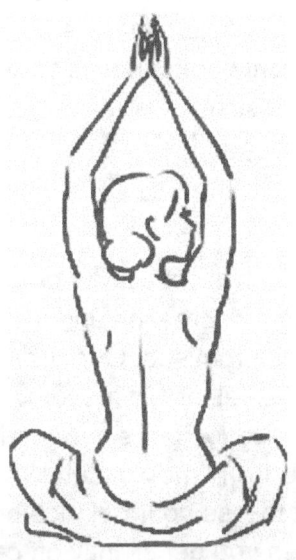

ALIGNMENT ~ PHASE 2

In the alignment phase, we focus on improving your posture, balance and overall stability. Before we start the exercise routine, let's look at why it's important to incorporate three different types of exercises to achieve alignment.

Posture, balance and stability work synergistically to keep your body in proper alignment. If you only focus on posture, you may still have issues with balance and stability. If you only focus on balance, your posture may still inhibit your recovery.

POSTURAL TRAINING:

Postural training is necessary to re-train your muscles to function properly and re-align the spinal column. Pain, guarding, and decreased self-confidence are conducive to postural changes. Your posture can improve, or it can hamper bodily functions and mobility. Improving your posture may also reduce chronic pain.

BALANCE:

The balance of the breast cancer survivor is often times affected. The loss of muscle mass and neuropathy (caused by some cytoxic medications) can lead to decreased proprioception, awareness of the position of your body. This can lead to a lack of balance.

STABILIZATION:

Due to reduced physical activity or lack of physical activity, your muscle strength decreases and the stability ofyou're your movements are compromised. Our core muscles (muscles of our trunk region) stabilize all of our movements.

Improving stabilization goes hand-in-hand with improving balance and efficiency in movement. When your core is strong, you are less likely to lose your balance because it's easier to catch yourself when you get slightly off center.

ALIGNMENT EXERCISES

POSTURAL TRAINING

Upper Back Strengthener

Exercise Check List

- Stand erect with your chin parallel to the ground.
- Relax your arms at your sides.
- Keep your abdominal muscles flexed.

Exercise Instructions

- Retract your neck muscles. This will pull your head straight back.
- It is important that you focus on your chin and keep it parallel to the ground.
- You will feel the muscles in the back of your neck working.

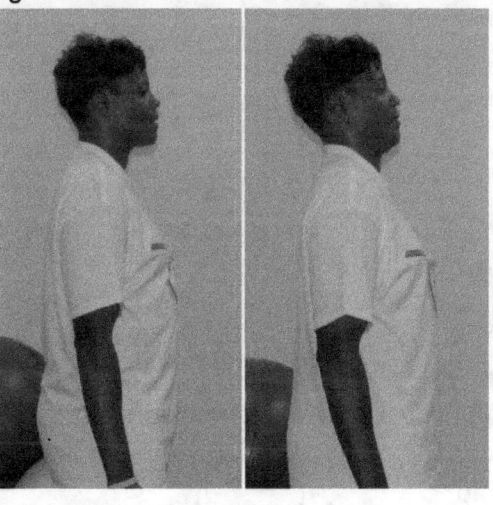

Progression as you grow stronger
1) 3 sets of 8 repetitions
2) 3 sets of 10 repetitions
3) 3 sets of 2 repetitions

Wall Angel

- Stand against a wall.
- Make sure your heels, your tailbone, elbows, wrists, shoulders and head are against the wall.
- Keep your chin parallel to the ground.
- Keep your abs tight. Your arms begin down at your side

- Begin to slowly raise your arms keeping your elbows, and wrists against the wall.

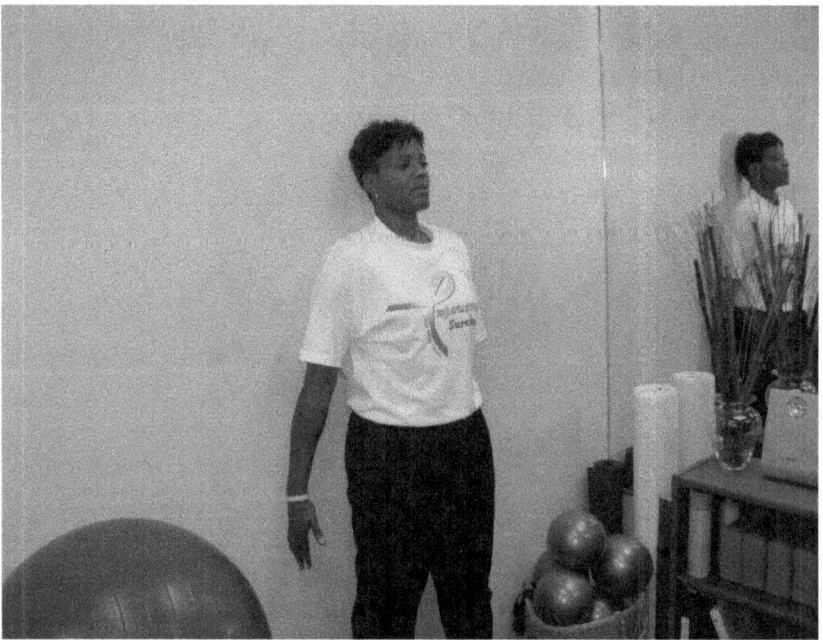

- Bring your arms as high as you can get them without pain. The goal is to bring your hands together above your head.
- Count it as one complete repetition when you have brought your hands as high as you can.

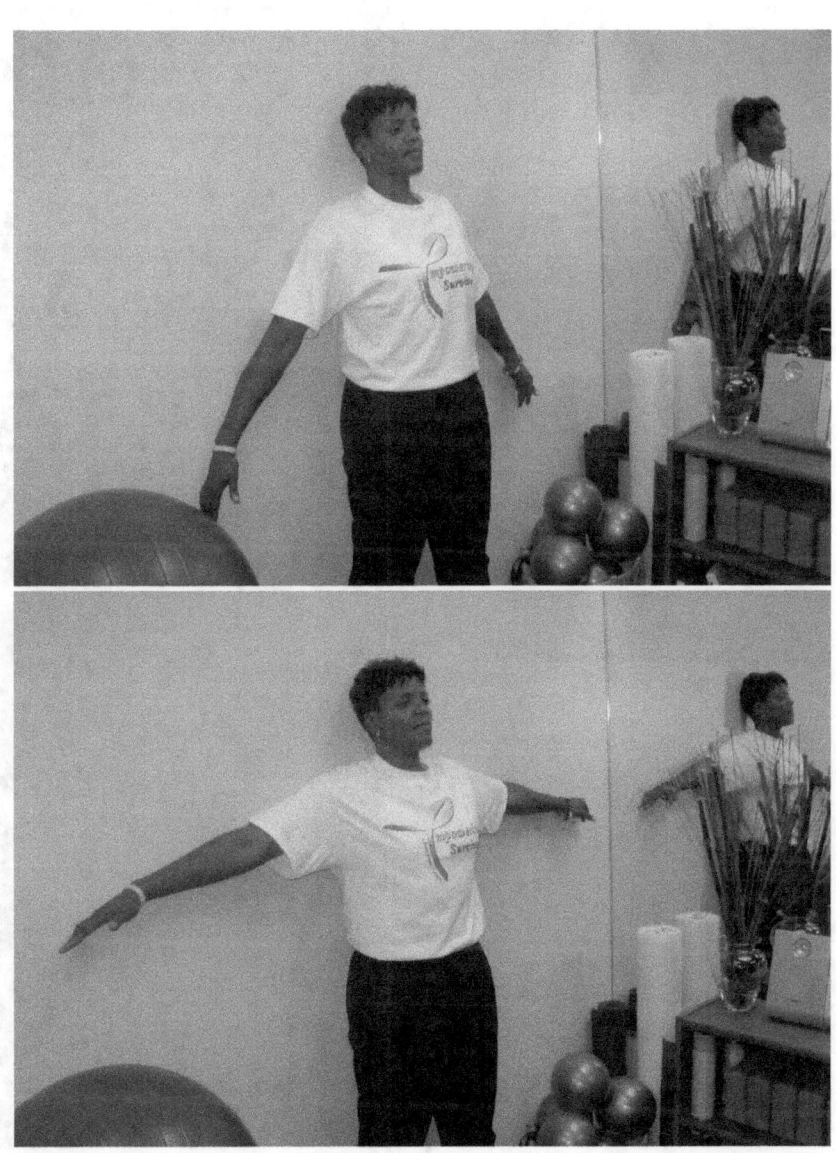

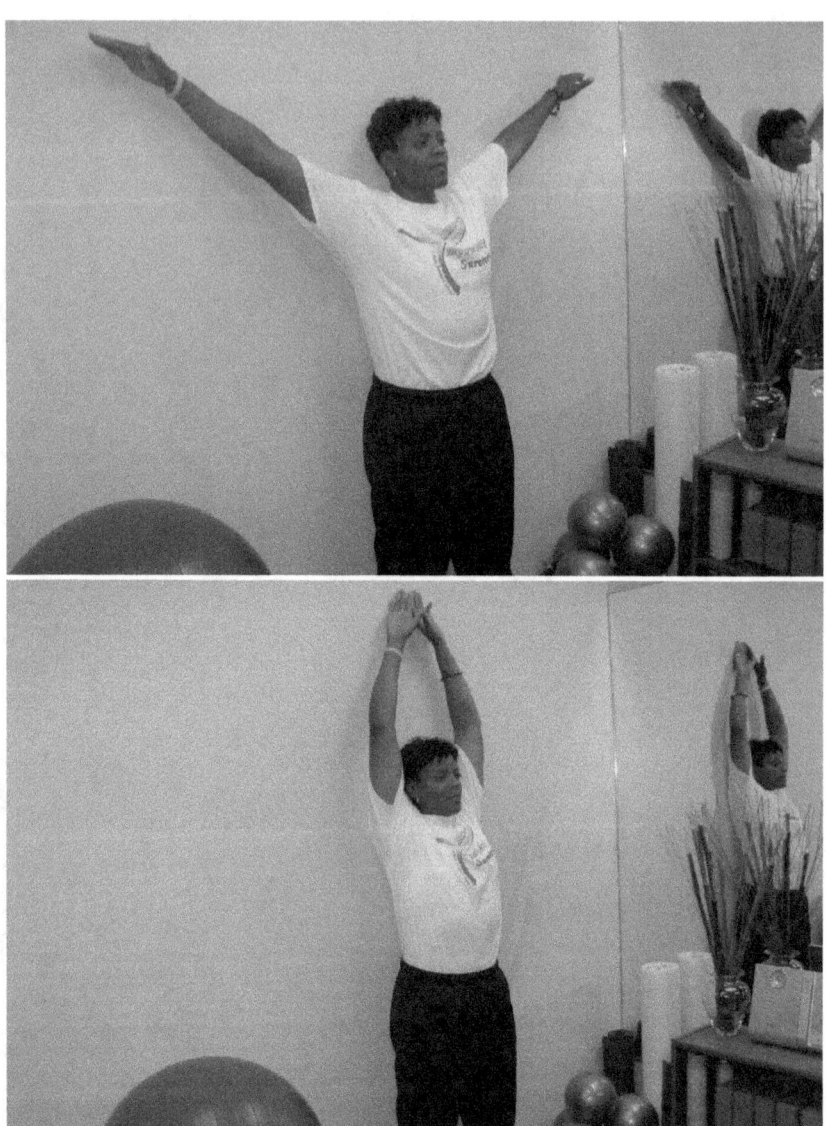

Progression as You Grow Stronger
1) 3 sets of 4-6 repetitions
2) 3 sets of 6-8 repetitions
3) 3 sets of 8-10.

BALANCE

One-Leg Stand

Exercise Check List
- Stand with your feet shoulder's width apart.
- Let you arms hang at your side.

Exercise Instructions
- Lift your right leg and hold it up while maintaining your balance.

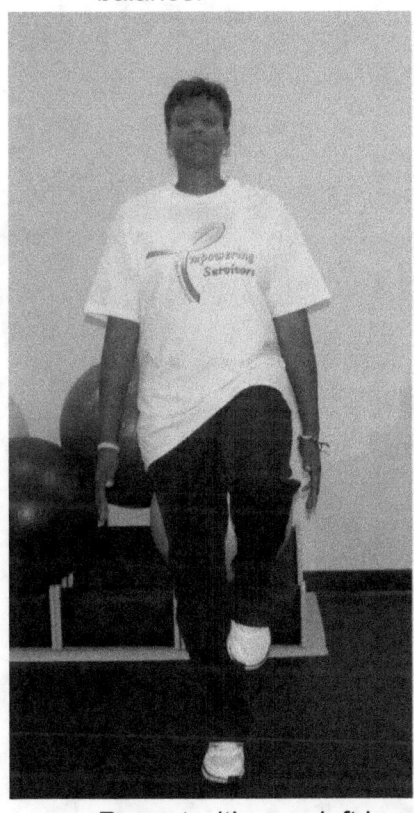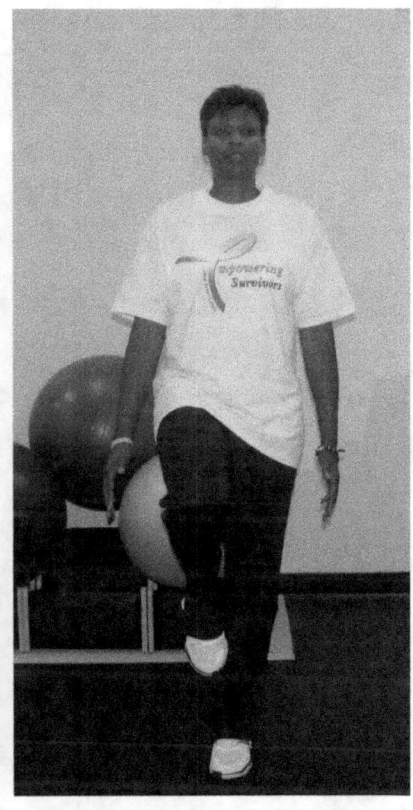

- Repeat with your left leg.

Progression as You Grow Stronger
1) 3 Sets of 10. Hold your balance for 10 seconds.
2) 3 Sets of 10. Hold your balance for 15 seconds
3) 3 Sets of 10. Hold your balance for 30 seconds

Note:

Perform one set on the right leg, then the left leg or alternate legs after each lift if this is more comfortable. Your goal is to hold 30 leg lifts on each side.

Staggered Stance

- Stand with your feet shoulder's width apart.
- Let you arms hang at your side.

Exercise Instructions
- Begin by stepping your right foot in front of your left foot.

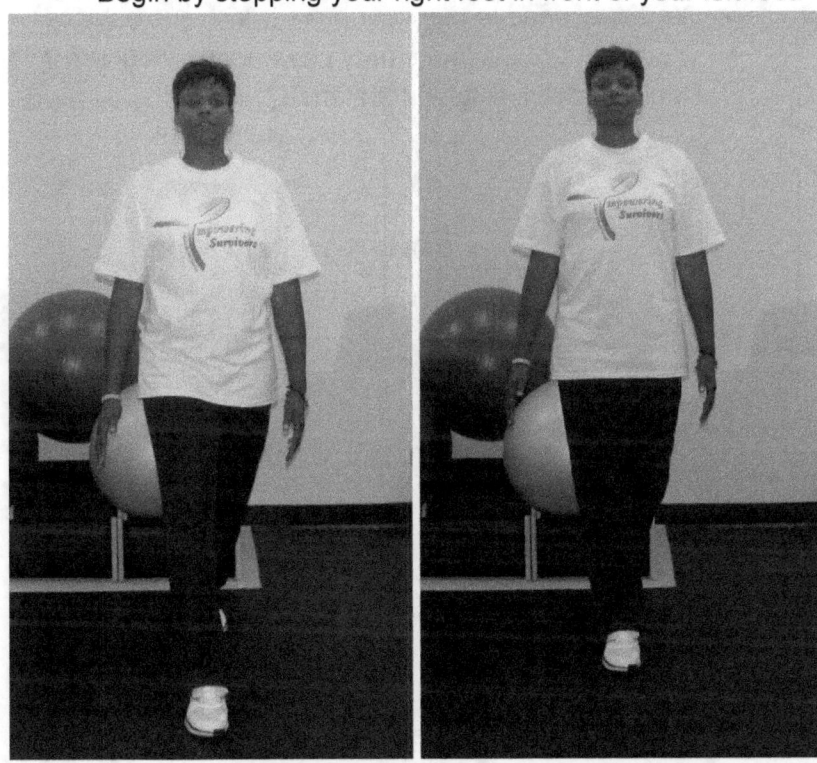

- Your right foot should be directly in front of your left foot as if you were walking a tight rope. The distance between the front and back foot should be approximately 12 inches.

Progression as You Grow Stronger
1) 3 Sets of 10. Hold your balance for 10 seconds.
2) 3 Sets of 10. Hold your balance for 15 seconds
3) 3 Sets of 10. Hold your balance for 30 seconds

Notes:

- As hold times get easier, take this as an indication that it is time to increase your hold times.
- As you get better at holding your balance, it's time to move on to the more advanced Heel-to-toe stance.
- Stand heel-to-toe with your right foot in front of your left foot. Hold your balance.
- You may need to use your arms to achieve balance.
- You can also place a sturdy chair nearby to grasp if you feel yourself losing your balance.

STABILITY EXERCISES

March on the Ball

You can begin by doing this exercise seated on a chair if you find it too difficult to balance on a ball.

Exercise Check List
- Sit balanced with your chin level to the ground.
- Keep your back straight.
- Place your feet approximately shoulder's width apart.
- Keep your abs tight.
- Your hands should be down at your sides.

Exercise Instructions
- Keeping your back straight and your abs tight, lift your right leg. Maintain balance.
- Then alternate and march with your left leg. Again, it is important to keep your chin level to the floor, your back straight and your stomach muscles tight.

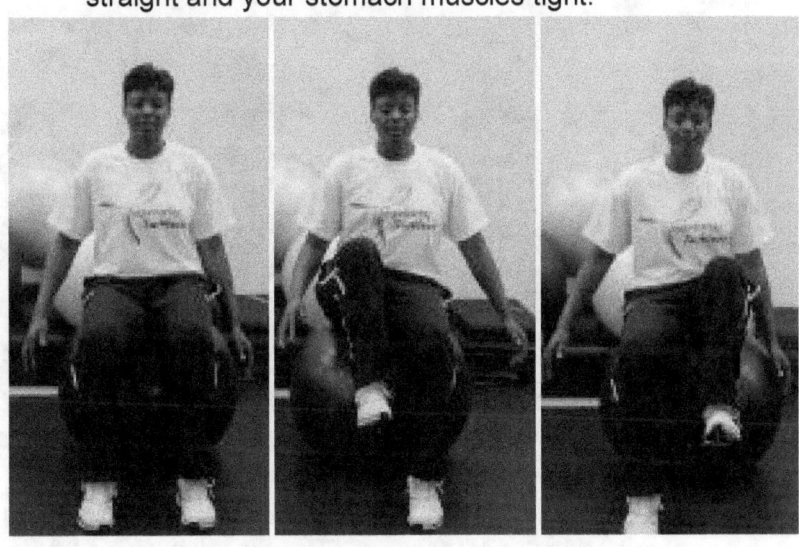

Progression as You Grow Stronger
1) 3 sets of 6-8 repetitions
2) 3 sets of 8-10 repetitions
3) 3 sets of 12-15 repetitions

Advanced March on the Ball

As you gain strength and endurance, marching with just your legs will become easy. This means it's time to advance to a more difficult version of Marching on the Ball.

Exercise Check List

- Sit balanced on the ball with your chin level to the ground, back straight and abs tight.
- Place your feet approximately shoulder's width apart.
- The key to maintaining control and balance as you perform the marching movement is keeping your mid-section contracted.

Exercise Instructions

- Keeping your back straight and your abs tight, lift your right leg and left arm. Inhale through the lift.

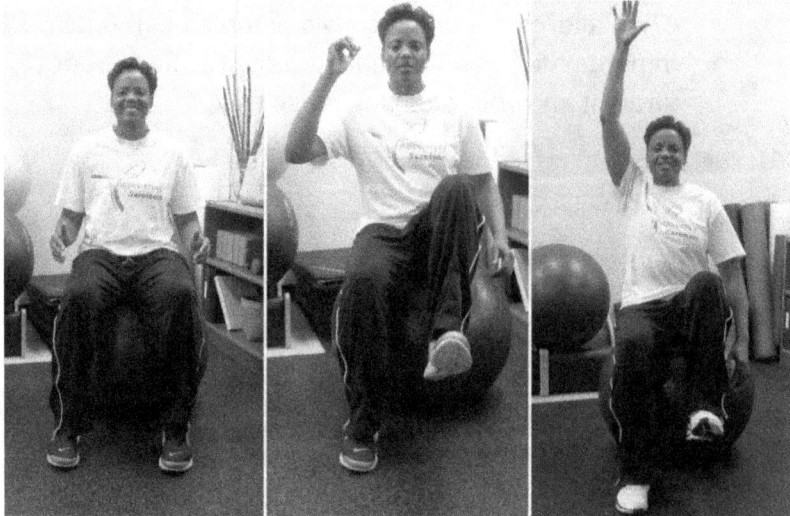

- Exhale as you lower your right leg and left arm and while you lift your left leg and lift your right arm.
- Continue alternating sides, breathing consciously until you have completed the number of repetitions for your fitness level.

Progression as You Grow Stronger
> 1) 3 sets of 6-8 repetitions
> 2) 3 sets of 8-10 repetitions
> 3) 3 sets of 12-15 repetitions

Notes:

Remember!!! Your chin stays level to the floor, your back stays straight, and your stomach muscles stay tight. Focus on staying balanced.

The Bridge

- Your shoulders, hips and knees should be in a straight line.
- Do not arch your back!
- Keep your abdominal muscles tight.

Exercise Instructions

- Lay on the ground with your knees bent.
- Your feet should be approximately shoulder's width apart. You may need to move your feet wider to maintain balance.
- Extend your arms down to your sides.

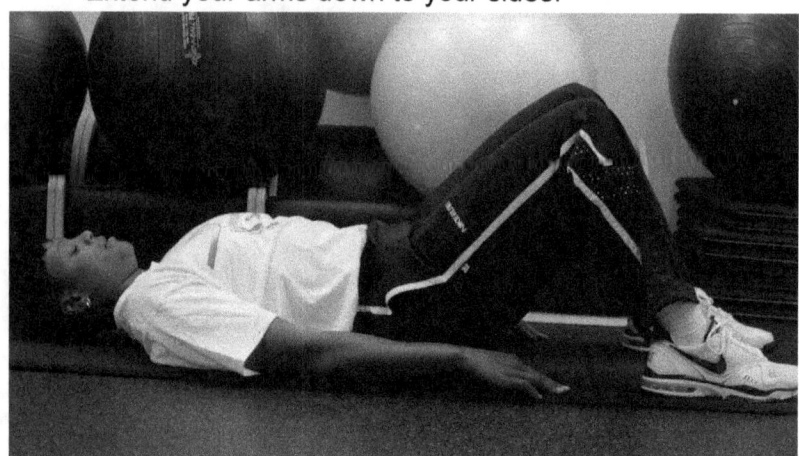

- Push through your heels, recruiting your hamstring and gluteus muscles to raise your hips off of the floor.

66

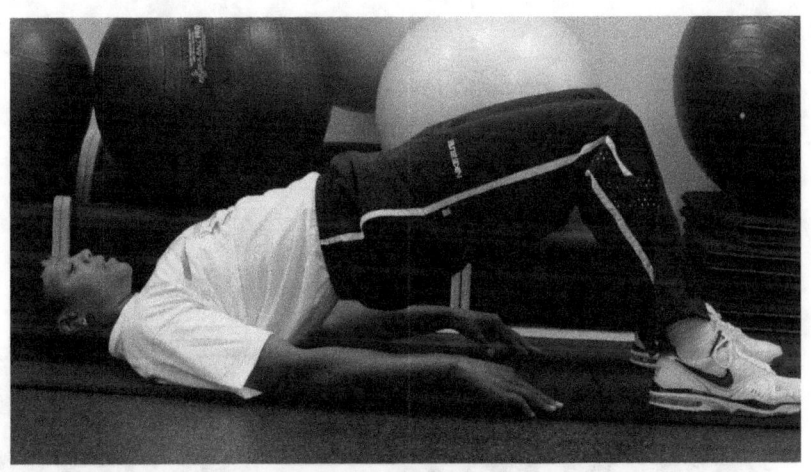

Progression as You Grow Stronger

1) 3 sets of 6-8 repetitions
2) 3 sets of 8-10 repetitions
3) 3 sets of 12-15 repetitions

Quadruped Position

This is a basic position for several exercises in this manual.
- Get down on the floor on your hands and knees.
- Place your wrists directly below your shoulders.
- Position your knees directly below your hips approximately shoulder's width apart.
- Align your body so you could draw a straight line from your tail bone to your head.

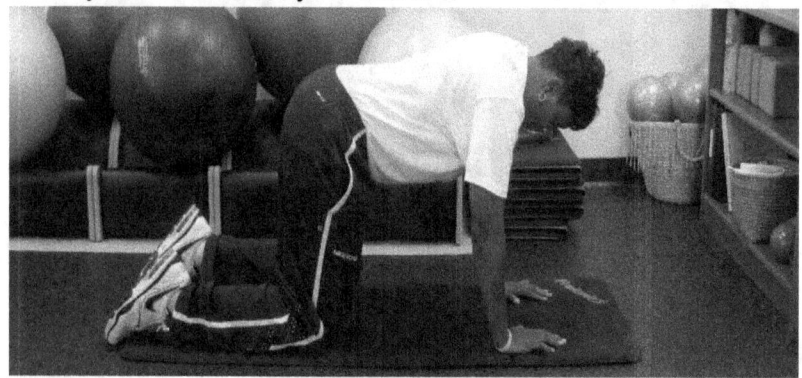

3-points Exercise

When the 3 points exercise no longer poses a challenge, advance to the *Two Points Exercise*.

Exercise Check List
- Keep your stomach muscles tight.
- Maintain your balance while extending your leg or arm.

Exercise Instructions
- Begin in the quadruped position where you have four points on the floor.
- Raise your left leg. Pretend you are kicking the wall behind you, and point your toes to the floor.
- Put your leg down.

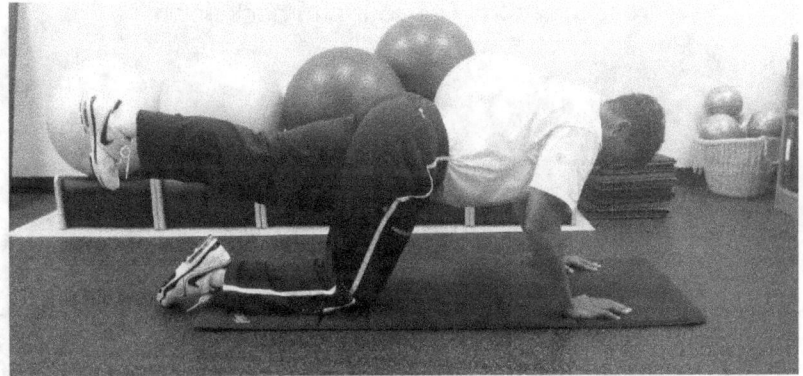

- Raise your right leg. Pretend you are kicking the wall behind you, and point your toes to the floor.

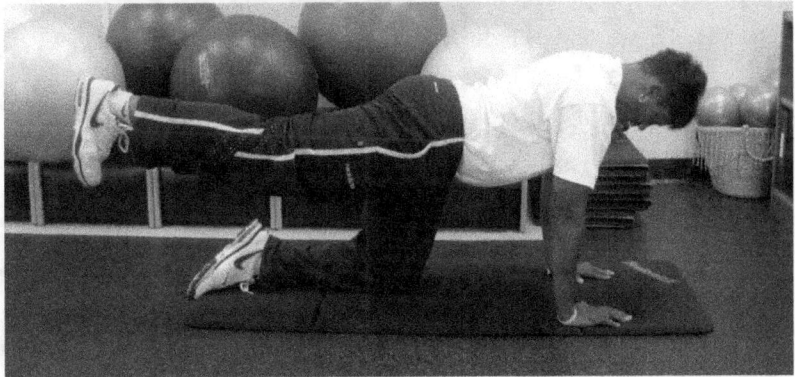

- Put your leg down.

- Raise your left arm. Pretend you are trying to reach across the room. Put your arm back down.

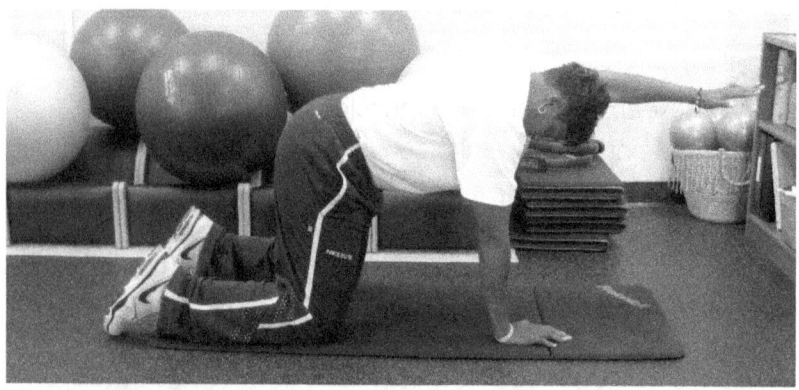

- Raise your right arm. Pretend you are trying to reach across the room. Put your arm back down.

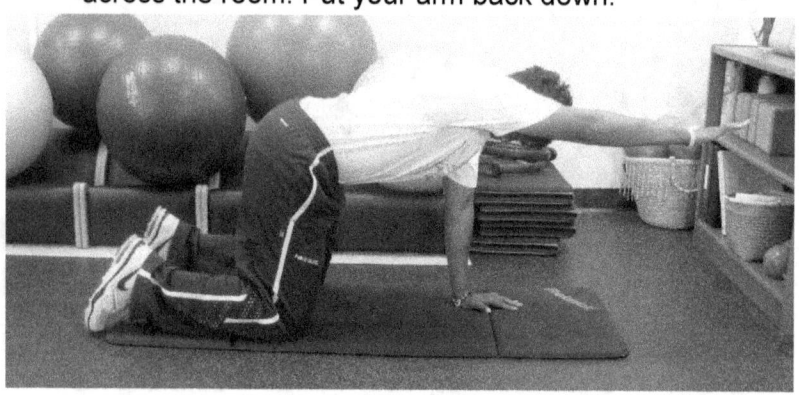

Progression as You Grow Stronger
1) 3 Sets of 10. Hold your balance for 10 seconds.
2) 3 Sets of 10. Hold your balance for 15 seconds
3) 3 Sets of 10. Hold your balance for 30 seconds

Two Points Exercise

- Keep your stomach muscles tight.
- Maintain your balance while extending your leg and arm.
- Imagine drawing a straight line from your heel to your fingers.

Exercise Instructions
- Begin in the quadruped position where you have four points on the floor.
- Extend your left arm and your right leg. Keeping your abdominal muscles tight,

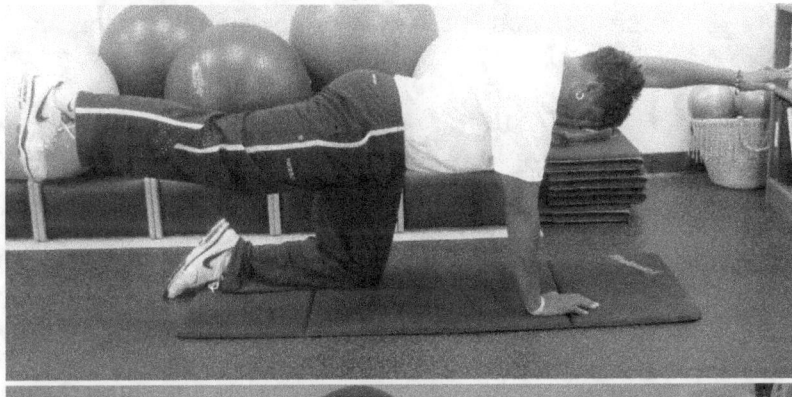

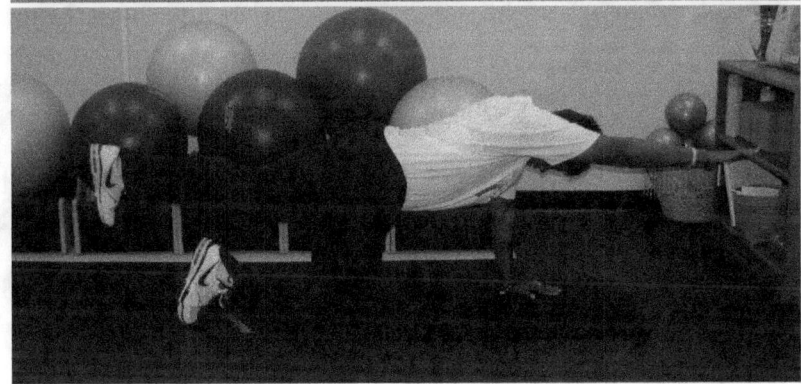

Progression as You Grow Stronger
1) 3 Sets of 10. Hold your balance for 10 seconds.
2) 3 Sets of 10. Hold your balance for 15 seconds
3) 3 Sets of 10. Hold your balance for 30 seconds

The Plank

Exercise Check List

- Find a level surface that will allow for foot traction.
- Look directly at the floor, keeping your spinal column in a straight line
- Make sure your elbows are situated directly under your shoulders and are shoulder's width apart.
- Your head should be level with your tail bone.
- Do not arch your back, and be sure your abdomen is tight.

Exercise Instructions

- Push your body up on your elbows and your toes.

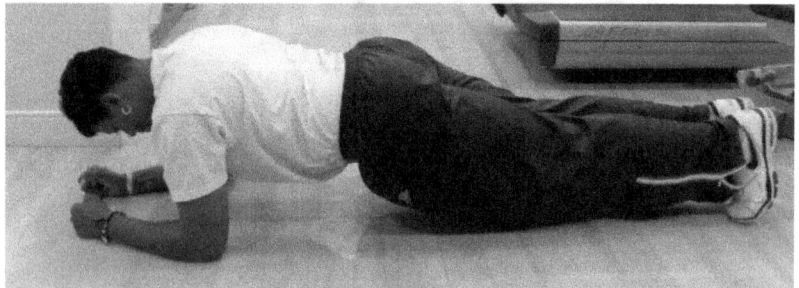

- Lift your left leg so your toe is about even with your heel.
- Hold as recommended (beginning with 8-10 seconds).
- Return to starting position.

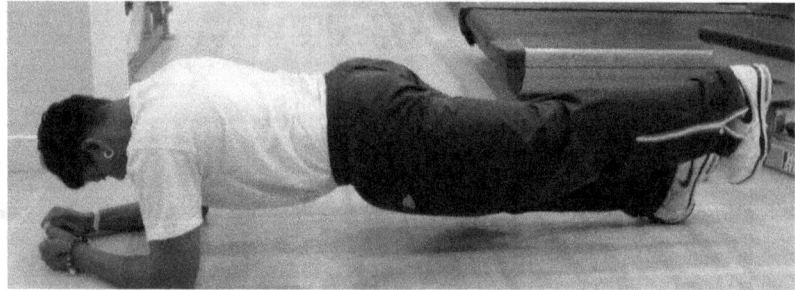

- Lift your right leg so your toe is even with your heel.
- Hold as recommended (beginning with 8-10 seconds).
- Return to starting position

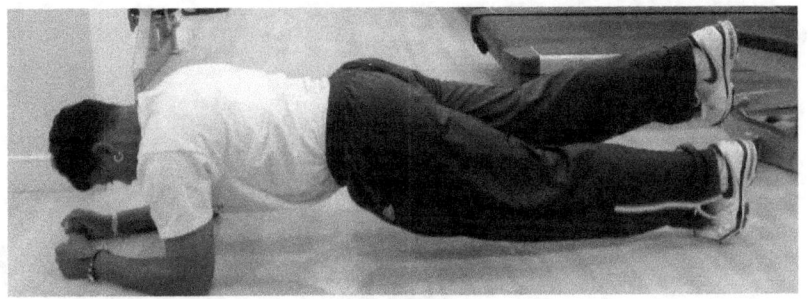

Progression as You Grow Stronger

   1) 3 sets with 8-10 second holds

   2) 3 sets with 12-15 second holds

   3) 3 sets of 15-20 second holds

You can increase the difficulty further by lifting your leg higher. Be careful not to arch the back if you do so.

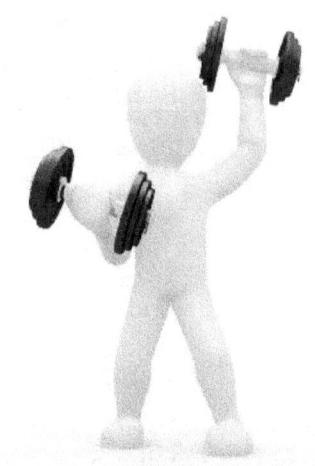

STRENGTH ~ PHASE 3

Now, you are ready to really power up. In Phase 2, you began to strengthen your core. Now, we're going to really focus on restoring your core to its full capacity.

We're also going to work on increasing another area of strength—functional strength. This is the strength you need to do all the activities you face in your daily life. For some of you, this may be more than for others, yet if you follow through with the exercises given here to increase your functional strength, you'll find yourself more capable, possibly more capable than you ever expected to be.

Finally, we're going to add the component of aerobic training. For many of you, working through the different phases may have left you feeling out of breath. If this is the case, you were getting a low level of aerobic exercise at that stage.

Of course, as you get stronger, you'll find that you have to do more to reach a point where you need to do more before you breath faster and get your heart pumping. That's when you are ready to start aerobic training in addition to your other exercises.

CORE STRENGTH:

Our core, or midsection, is where all of our movement originates. Decreased activity levels, and muscle atrophy result in a reduction in core strength. To achieve long-term strength, the core needs to come first.

FUNCTIONAL STRENGTH:

Improving functional strength will directly increase your quality of living. Ultimately this program has been designed to do just that.

Functional strength is the strength you need to be functional in your day-to-day life. Being able to get dressed, climb stairs, put groceries away are all activities we take for granted until we don't have the ability to perform them. The focus of this component is exercising to improve strength that will transfer to and facilitate your everyday activities.

AEROBIC TRAINING:

Your ability to sustain exercise over a period of time has probably been diminished as a result of your surgery and subsequent treatment regimens. The overall treatment process takes a toll on your body system as a whole. It decreases our ability to exert ourselves continuously over time.

Conditioning the body in this way improves your lung capacity, contributes to your cardiovascular health, improves your muscle tone and promotes weight loss.

STRENGTH BUILDING EXERCISES

CORE EXERCISES

Bicycle – Beginner's Level

Exercise Check List

- Keep the small of your back pressed to the floor. Do not arch your back.
- Make sure your head and shoulders stay on the ground.
- Place your hands under your buttocks to support your lower back.
- Keep your abdominal muscles tight.

Exercise Instructions

- Lay flat on the floor.
- Bend your knees, bringing them toward your chest until they are above your hips.
- Visualize yourself riding a bike.
- Start moving your legs in that motion.

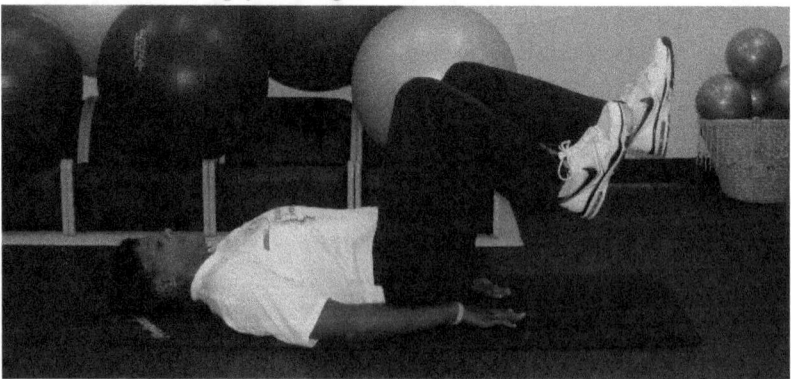

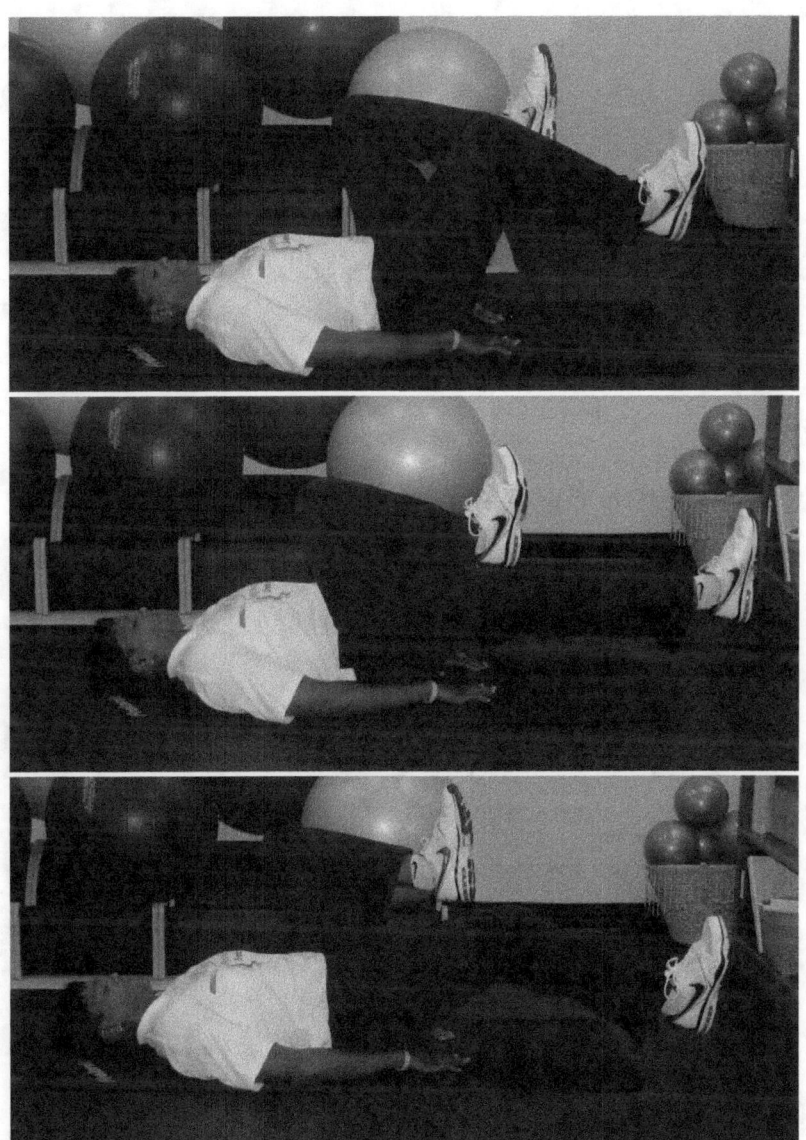

Progression as You Grow Stronger

1) 3 Sets of 5-7 pedals for each leg.
2) 3 Sets of 8-10 pedals for each leg.
3) 3 Sets of 12-15 pedals for each leg.

Bicycle – Advanced Level

Rising up onto your elbows will increase the difficulty of the bicycle exercise.

Exercise Check List

- Be sure to keep your elbows directly below your shoulders, and do not arch your back.
- Keep your abdominal muscles tight.
- Move your feet as if you are riding a bike.

Exercise Instructions

- Bend your right knee.
- Lift your feet off the floor.
- Visualize yourself riding a bike.
- Alternate bringing your right leg up and pushing your left leg straight, then pulling your left leg up and pushing your right leg straight.

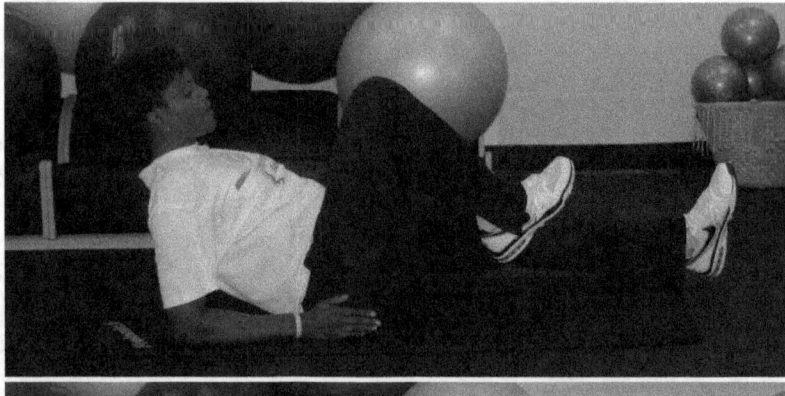

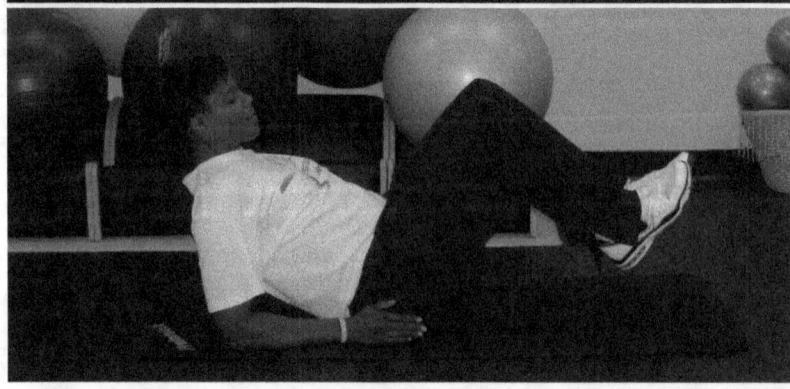

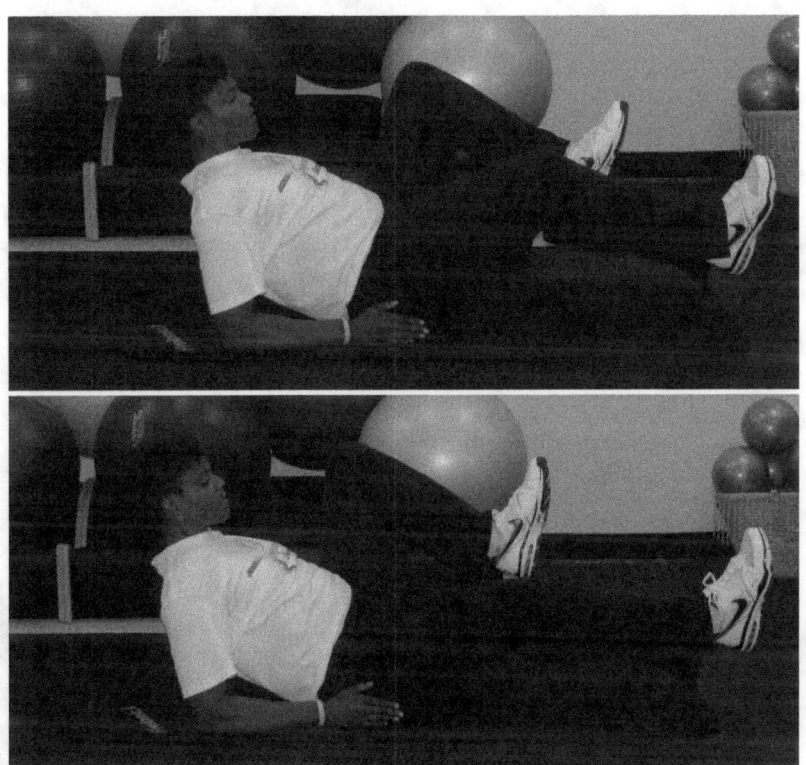

Progression as You Grow Stronger

1) 3 Sets of 5-7 pedals for each leg.
2) 3 Sets of 8-10 pedals for each leg.
3) 3 Sets of 12-15 pedals for each leg.

Balance Ball

Exercise Check List

- Get balanced with the exercise ball just below your shoulder blades.
- Make sure you maintain a straight line from your head to your knees.
- Tighten your abdominal muscles.
- Positions your feet approximately shoulder's width apart.

Exercise Instructions

- Looking up to the ceiling, extend both arms.

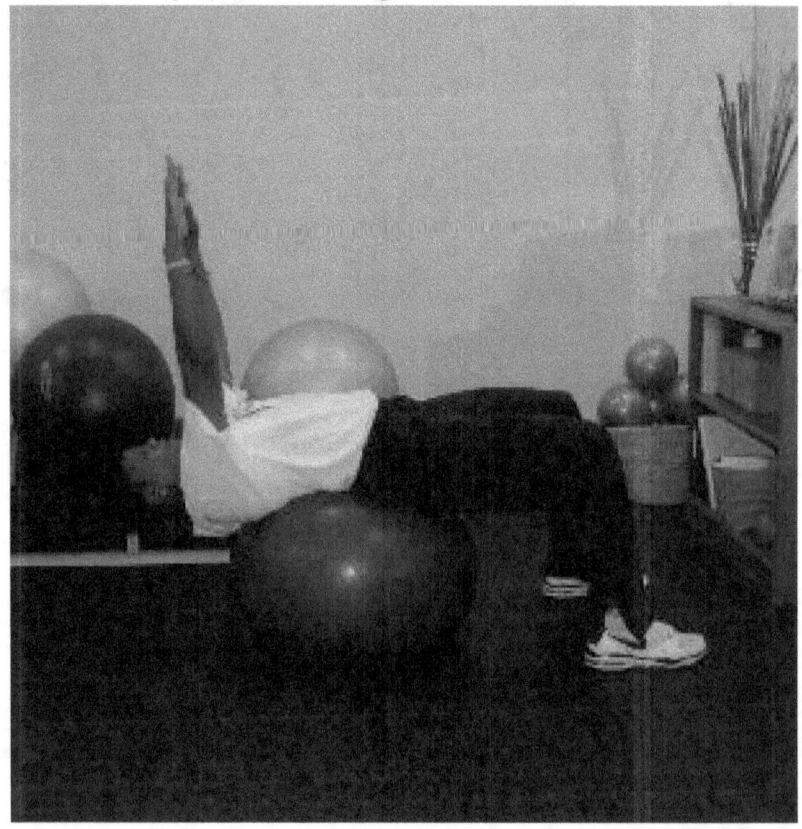

- Keep your eyes focused on the ceiling, and arms extended. Your stomach muscles must remain tight as you roll your spine off of the ball.

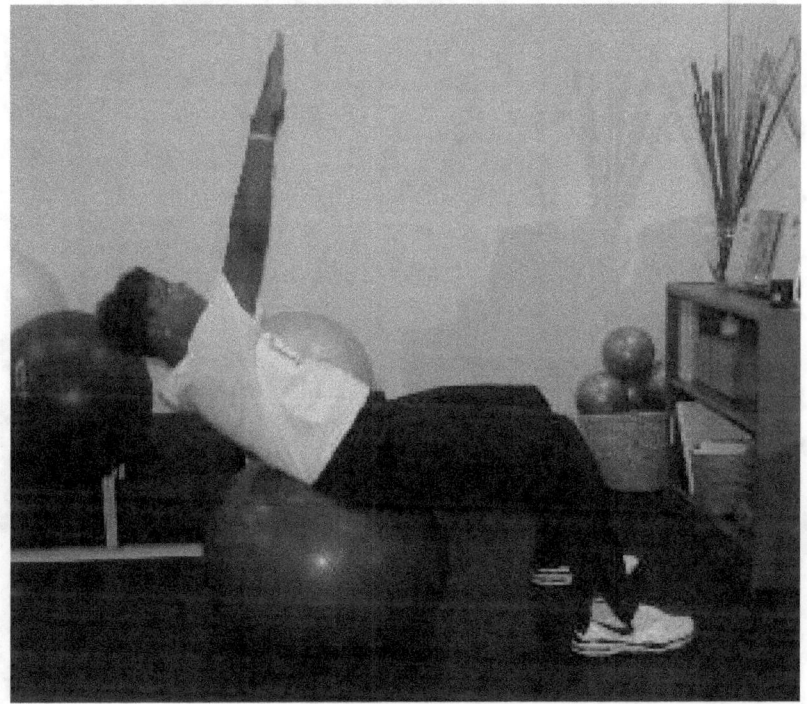

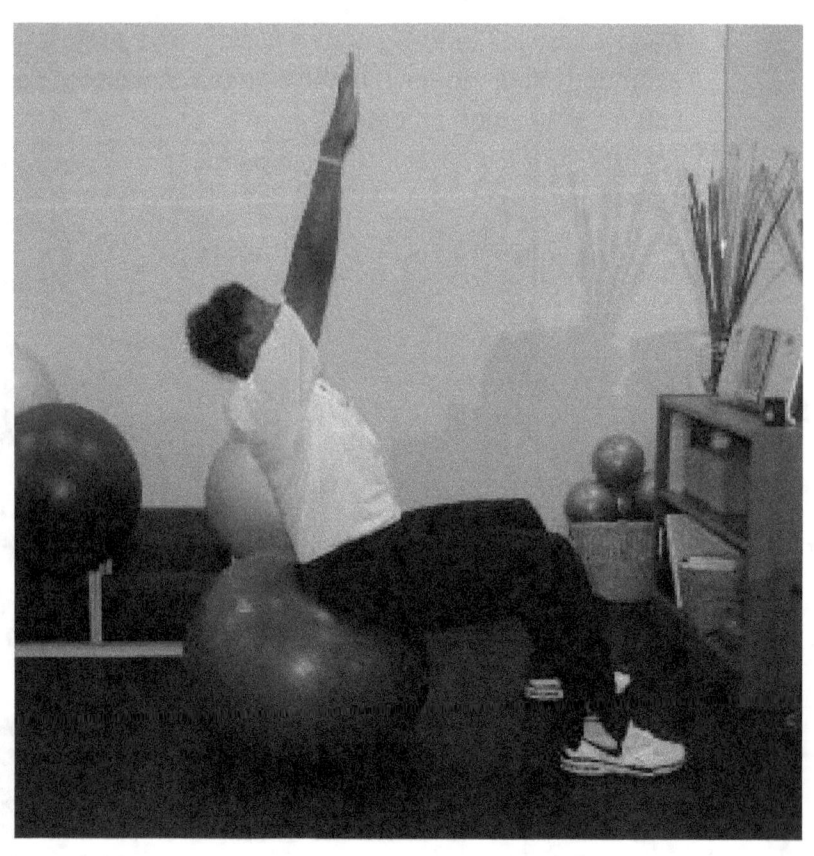

- Roll up until your back is straight.

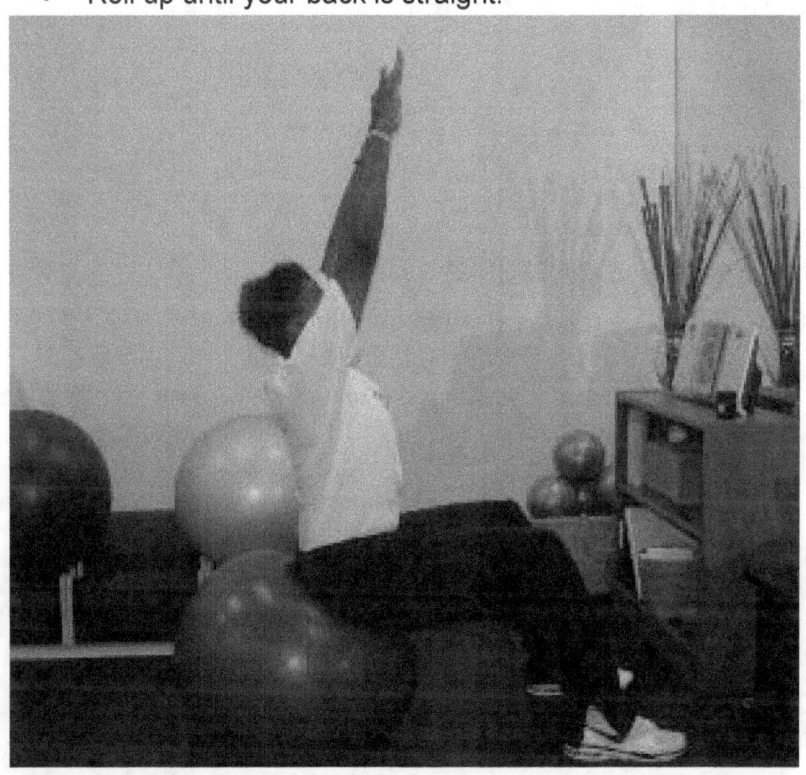

Progression as You Grow Stronger
1) 3 sets of 6-8 repetitions
2) 3 sets of 8-10 repetitions
3) 3 sets of 12-15 repetitions

FUNCTIONAL STRENGTH

Front Step-Ups

You will use a step or a box for this exercise.

Exercise Check List
- Stand with your chin level to the floor.
- Place feet shoulder's width apart.
- Keep your back straight.
- Hold your abdominal muscles tight.
- Keep your knee aligned with you ankle as you step up.

Exercise Instructions
- Step up with your right leg. (Make sure your knee does not go over your toes.)
- Raise your left knee and right arm.

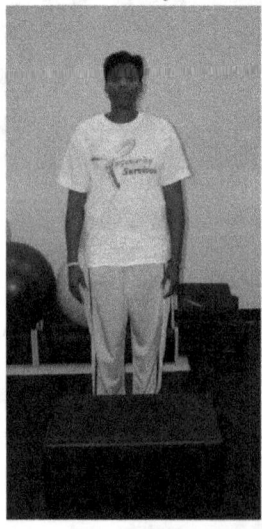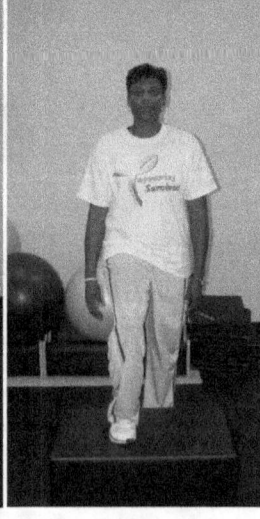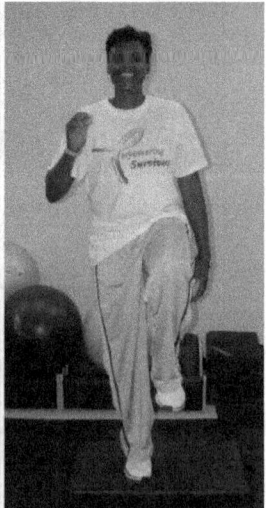

- Step back down to the floor.
- Alternate the leg you step up with.

Progression as You Grow Stronger
1) 3 sets of 8-10 for each leg.
2) 3 sets of 10-12 for each leg.
3) 3 sets of 12-15 for each leg.

<u>Step-Up From The Right Side</u>

You will use a step or a box for this exercise.

- Stand with your chin level to the floor.
- Place feet shoulder's width apart.
- Keep your back straight.
- Hold your abdominal muscles tight.
- Keep your knee aligned with you ankle as you step.

- Begin with your box or step to your right.
- Step up onto the box or step with your right leg.
- Raise your left knee and right arm.

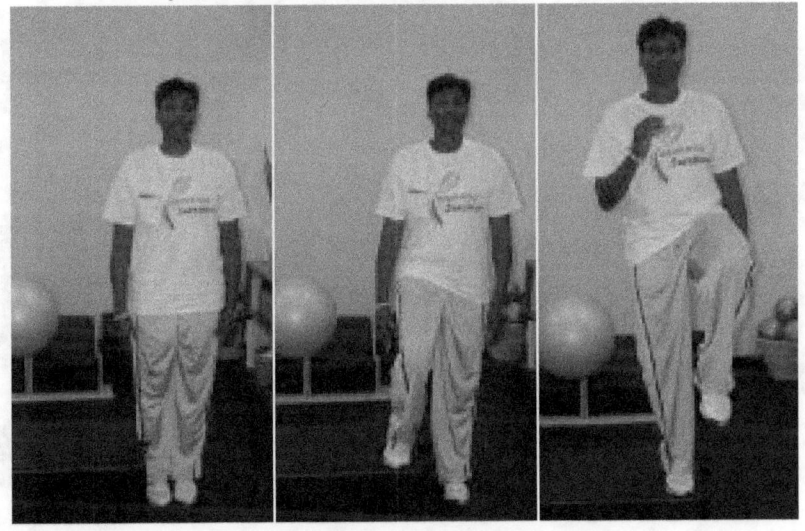

1) 3 sets of 8-10 for each leg.
2) 3 sets of 10-12 for each leg.
3) 3 sets of 12-15 for each leg.

Step-Up From The Left Side

You will use a step or a box for this exercise.

Exercise Check List

- Stand with your chin level to the floor.
- Place feet shoulder's width apart.
- Keep your back straight.
- Hold your abdominal muscles tight.
- Keep your knee aligned with you ankle as you step.

Exercise Instructions

- Begin with your box or step to your left.
- Step up onto the box or step with your right leg.
- Raise your right knee and your left arm at the same time.

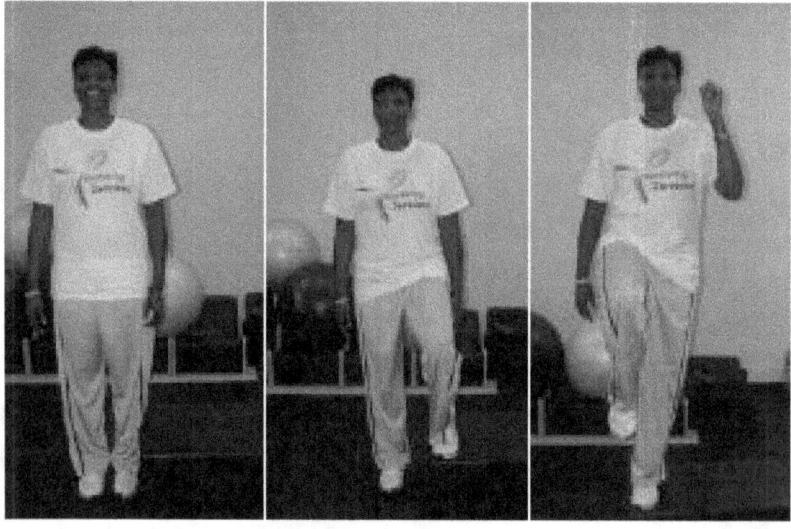

Progression as You Grow Stronger

1) 3 sets of 8-10 for each leg.
2) 3 sets of 10-12 for each leg.
3) 3 sets of 12-15 for each leg.

Wall Pumps

- Keep your back straight.
- Hold your abdominal muscles tight.
- Place your feet shoulder's width apart.

Exercise Instructions

- Stand facing the wall, approximately 1 foot from a wall.
- Place hands flat against the wall.
- Lean forward with your elbows extended.
- Slowly bend your arms allowing your body to move closer to the wall.
- Stop when you get as close to the wall as you can without touching it with your head or chest.
- Push yourself away from the wall. That is one pump.

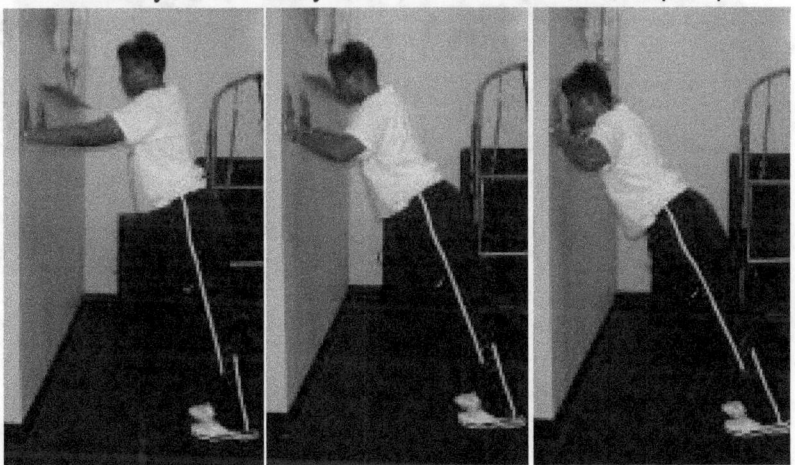

Progression as You Grow Stronger

1) 3 sets of 5-7 pumps.
2) 3 sets of 8-10 pumps.
3) 3 sets of 12-15 pumps.

Notes:

As you grow stronger, move your feet farther from the wall. Then switch to using the counter top instead of the wall.

87

<u>*Modified Pump*</u>

As you gain strength, you can progress to the modified pump and omit the wall pump.

Exercise Check List

- Do not arch your back. It should be in a straight line from your knees to your head.
- Keep your abs tight.
- Position your wrists directly below your shoulders.

Exercise Instructions

- Begin on your knees and the palms of your hands.
- Cross your ankles and lift your feet off of the floor.

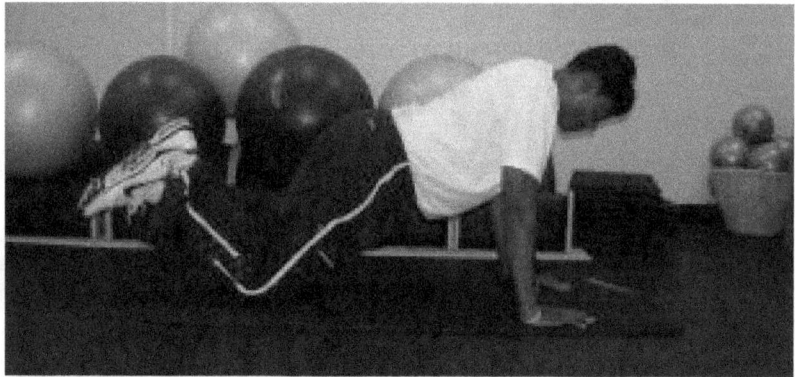

- Lower yourself to the floor.

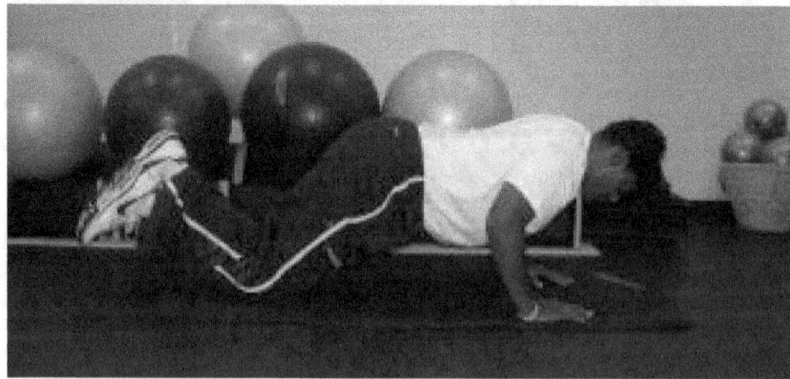

- Down to the floor and back up is one push-up.

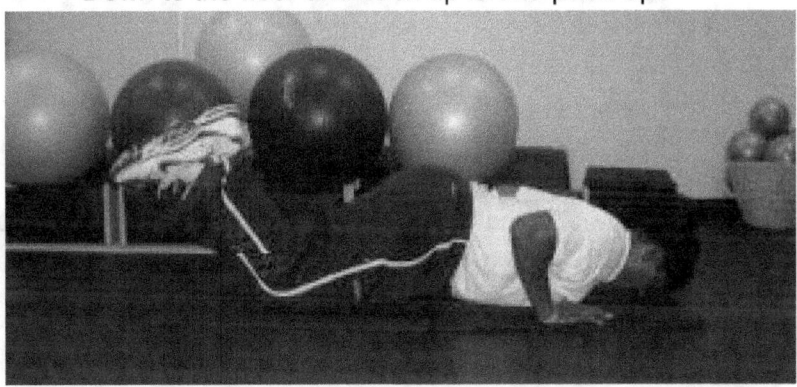

Progression as You Grow Stronger
1) 3 sets of 5-7 pumps.
2) 3 sets of 8-10 pumps.
3) 3 sets of 12-15 pumps.

AEROBIC TRAINING EXERCISES

Aerobic training can be achieved with a variety of exercise types— walking, running, bicycling, or using a treadmill. The key to this type of training is keeping your heart rate within 65-75% of your maximum heart rate.

Calculating Your Target Heart Rate

First, you will need to know how to calculate you maximum heart rate. To do this, you subtract your age from 220. For instance, if you are 25 years of age, you will subtract 25 from 220. That equals 195. 195 is your maximum heart rate.

Next you must determine your aerobic training zone. You calculate 65% of 195 by multiplying 195 by 0.65. That equals 127. 75% of 195 is calculated by multiplying 195 by 0.75. That equals 146.

All numbers are rounded to nearest whole number. So your target aerobic training zone would be a heart rate between 127 and 146.

Some equipment you use will have the ability to calculate heart rate. Otherwise, you can use a heart rate monitor or take your pulse manually.

The easiest way to get your heart rate is to calculate your radial pulse. This is done by taking your index finger and your middle finger and applying them LIGHTLY to the small indentation below the thumb on your opposite hand. Count your pulse for 15 seconds and multiply by 4, or count your pulse for 30 seconds and multiply by 2.

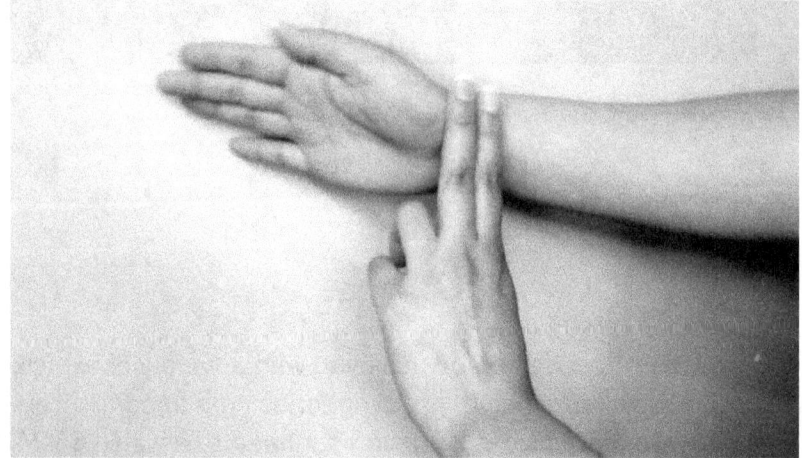

Now, that you've calculated what your heart rate should be, choose the exercise that you most enjoy. Do anything that gets your heart rate into the target range without leaving you feeling exhausted.

Walking is a great exercise to start with. It's easy on the joints and less likely to leave you discouraged. It's a good starting point if your goal is to run.

There are plenty of exercise machines available to get started with as well. Treadmills, elliptical trainers, bicycles, stepping machines, etc. These are all machines designed to support aerobic benefits.

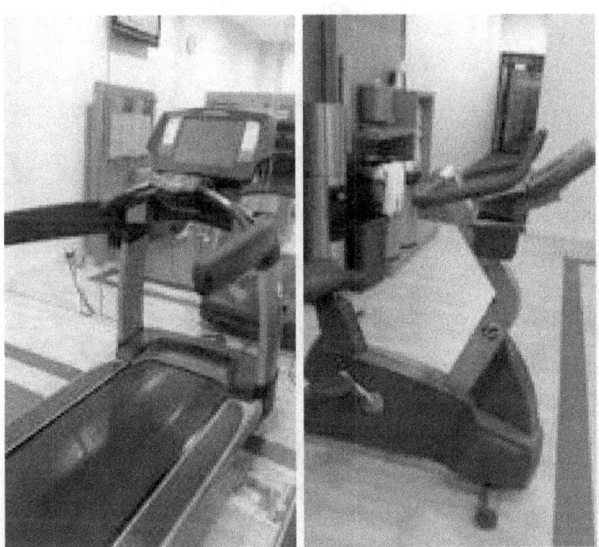

As a basic piece of equipment, the treadmill is a really good choice. You can use a treadmill to increase your fitness level gradually, and you are less likely to become frustrated with it.

Begin with the level flat and at a slow enough speed that you can sustain your target heart rate for 20 to 30 minutes. You can even start with 10 minute sessions and work your way up to longer sessions.

Science has proven that you don't have to exercise for 30 minutes at a time to experience aerobic benefits. Three 10 minutes quick-burst sessions where you spend about 2 minutes at a warm-up speed, then increase the intensity to the top of your target heart zone for about six minutes before cooling down at a slower pace again will help you increase your aerobic capacity quickly. These three burst sessions work just as well if you space them out over the day as if you do all three in one session.

In fact, there is some evidence that your body actually benefits more from micro exercise sessions that prolonged exercise sessions. It appears that the rest between sessions actually helps your body repair itself more efficiently, leading to less fatigue.

That's a trick that we breast cancer survivors can use!

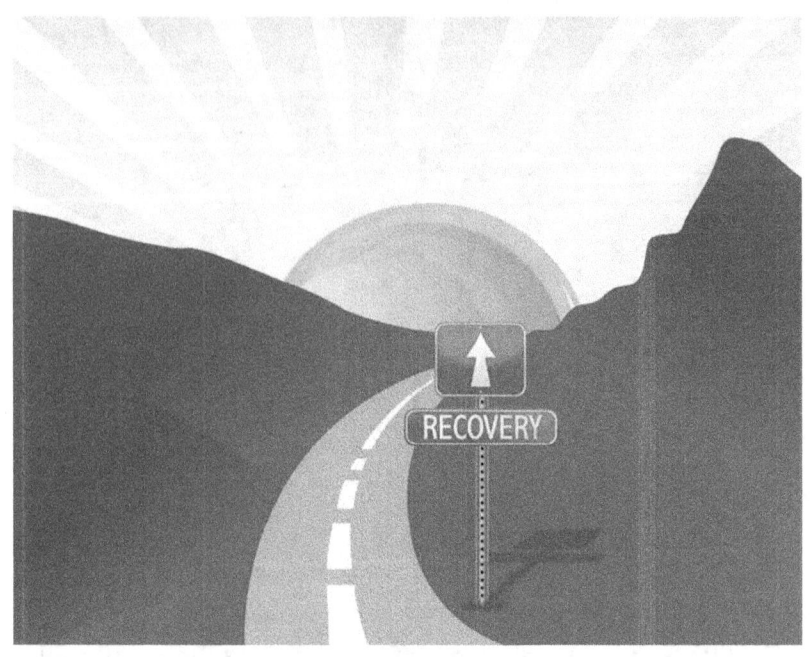

PERSONALIZED EXERCISE ~ PHASE 4

PERSONALIZED STRENGTH AND CONDITIONING:

This level of the recovery exercise program uses the previous phases as a foundation. Overall health is rooted in a consistent, total body, personalized fitness program.

<u>*Bench Press*</u>

This exercise can be done on an exercise bench or on a physio-ball as shown here.

Exercise Check List

- Your body should be balanced with the physio-ball under your shoulder blades.
- Your hips, knees, and shoulders should be in a straight line.
- Keep your abdomen tight.

Exercise Instructions

- Begin with dumbbells in each hand, forearms parallel to the floor and hands at right angle toward the ceiling.

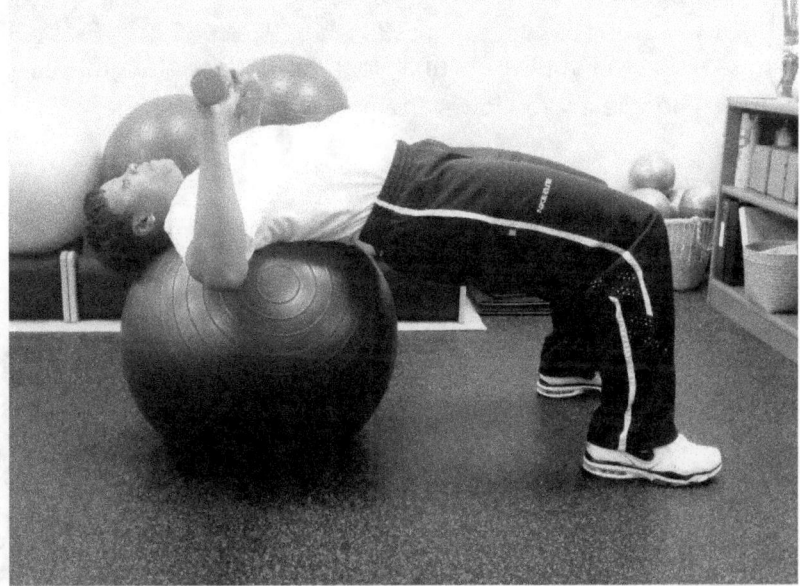

- Exhale while raising the dumbbells.
- Raise the dumbbells above your body directly over your chest.

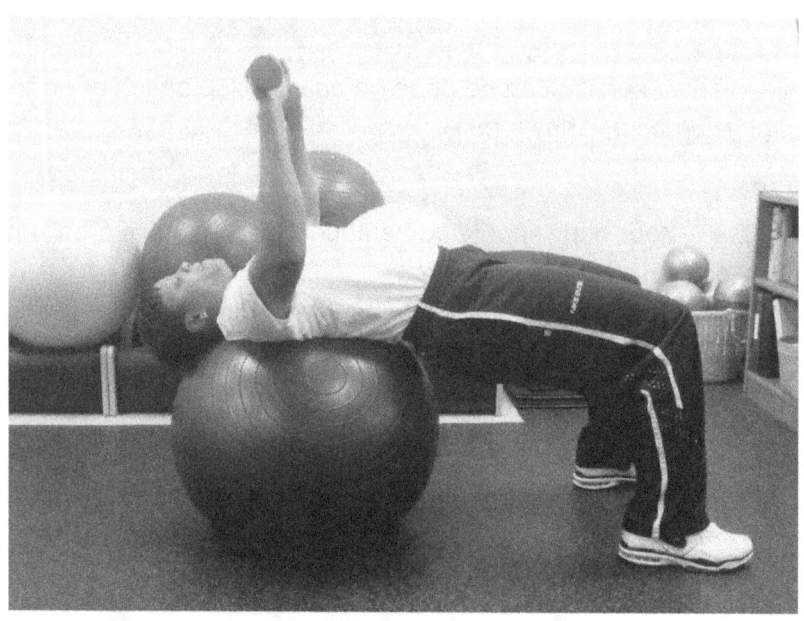

- Extend your arms until your elbows are straight.
- Inhale as you lower them.

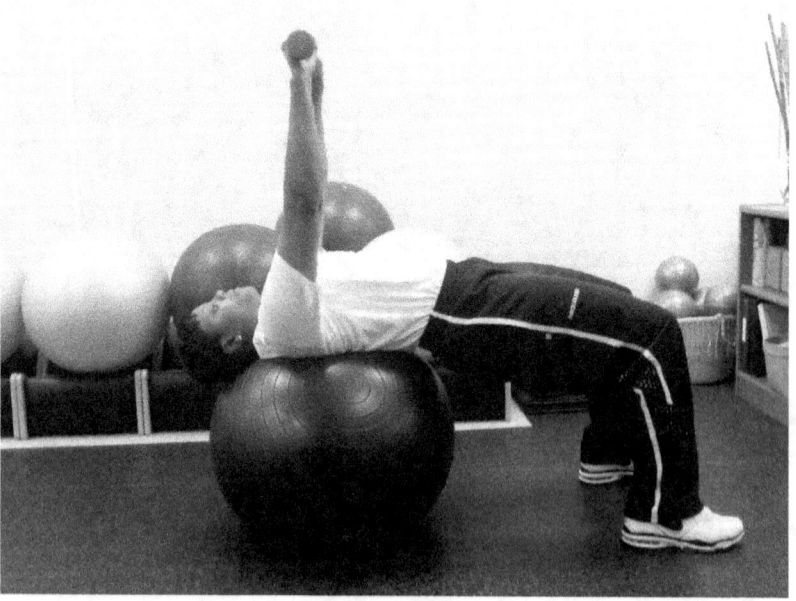

Progression as You Grow Stronger
1) 3 sets 8-10 repetitions
2) 3 sets 10-12 receptions
3) 3 sets of 12- 15 repetitions

Two-Arm Dumbbell Rows

Exercise Check List

- Bend knees slightly.
- Bend forward from the hip, allowing a slight arch in your lower back. You don't want to round the back toward the ceiling.
- Keep your abdomen tight. This will support your back.
- Keep hands facing to the inside.
- Do the exercise slowly, without jerking.

Exercise Instructions

- Hold a weight in each hand with your arms straight at your side.
- Lift the weight to your waist, bringing your elbow up until the back of your arm is as high as it is comfortable to raise it.
- Slowly lower the weights back down to your sides.

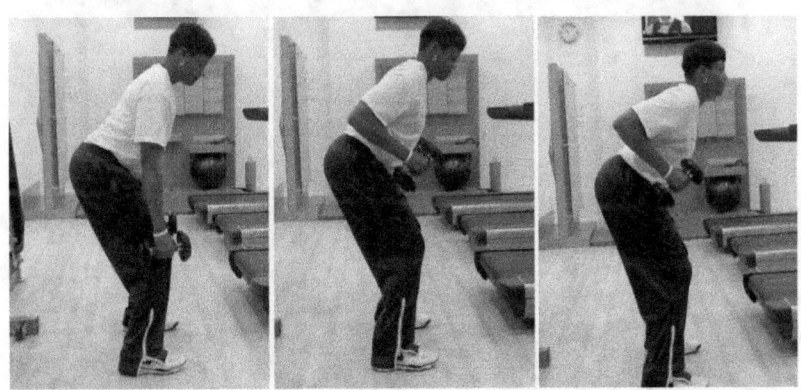

Progression as You Grow Stronger

1) 3 sets 8-10 repetitions
2) 3 sets 10-12 receptions
3) 3 sets of 12- 15 repetitions

Increase the weight of the dumbbells as you grow stronger. You may begin with one pound and increase weight as you are able.

Back Extension

Exercise Check List
- Your ribs and hips should be centered on the ball.
- Keep your abdomen tight.

Exercise Instructions
- Balance your body while lying face down on a physio-ball.
- Extend your arm out a 45 degree angle from your body.

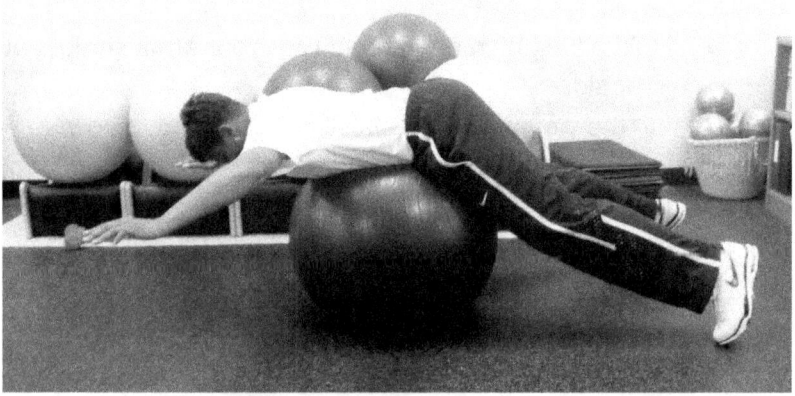

- Raise your torso up off the ball.

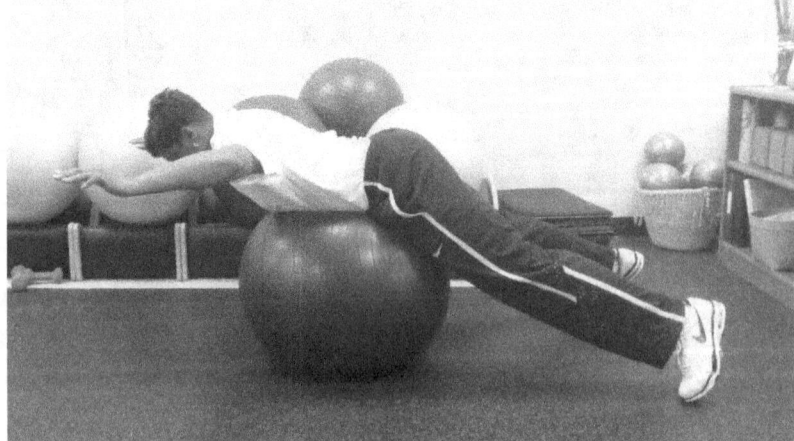

- The repetition is complete when your body is in a straight line.

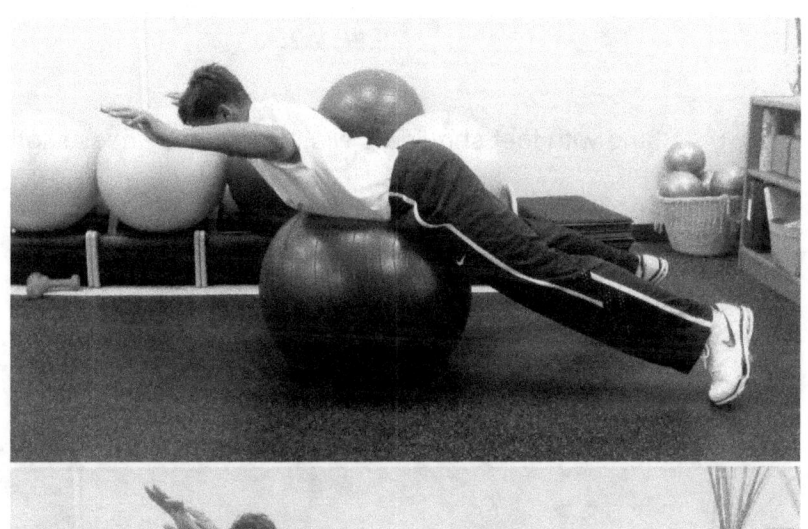

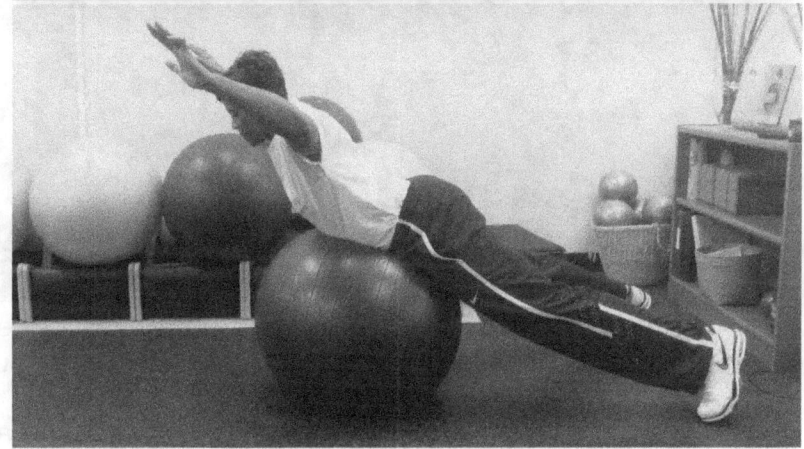

Progression as You Grow Stronger
1) 3 sets of 6-8 repetitions
2) 3 sets of 8-10 repetitions
3) 3 sets of 10-12 repetitions

Bicep Curl

- Stand with feet shoulders width apart and knees sligthly bent.
- Keep your head up, your back straight, and abdominals contracted.
- Allow the hand weights to hang at your side with the inside of your hand facing your body.

Exercise Instructions

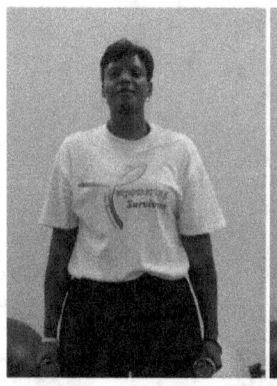 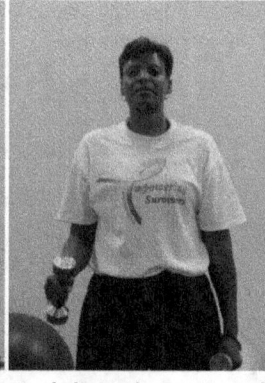 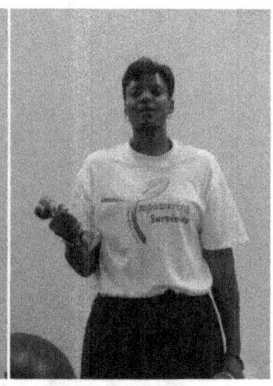

- Raise your right hand, keeping your elbow at your side.
- As you perform the bicep curl, turn your fist so that your fist faces your shoulder.
- The curl is complete when you cannot move your fist any closer to your shoulder.

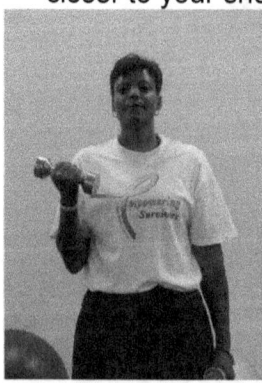 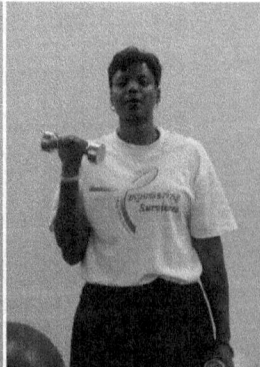 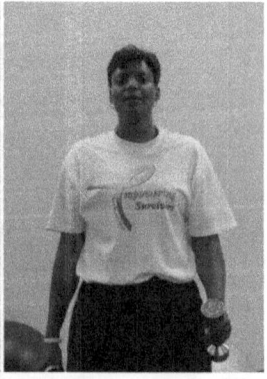

- Lower your arm back to your side, reversing the motion so your hand faces your side at the hip.

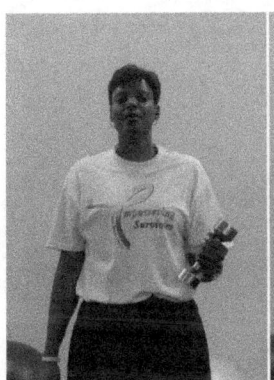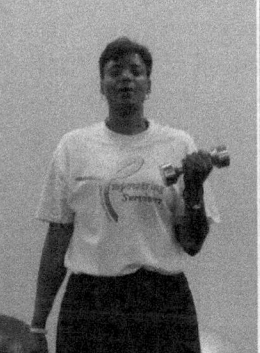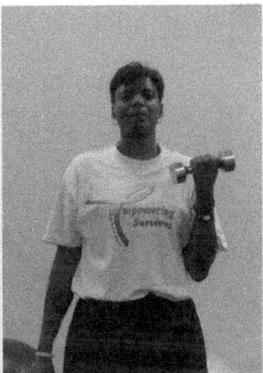

- Repeat the exercise with your left arm.

Progression as You Grow Stronger
1) 3 sets of 8-10 repetitions
2) 3 sets of 10-12 repetitions
3) 3 sets of 12-15 repetitions

Triceps Kick-back

Use a physio-ball or chair for this exercise.

Exercise Check List
- From your shoulder to your elbow your arm should be level with your back.
- Your head, shoulders and hips should be in a straight line.

Exercise Instructions
- Bend forward and look at the floor.
- Bend your knees slightly, and support your body weight with your left hand resting on the exercise ball.
- Hold a dumbbell in your right hand.
- Bend your elbow at a 90 degree angle.

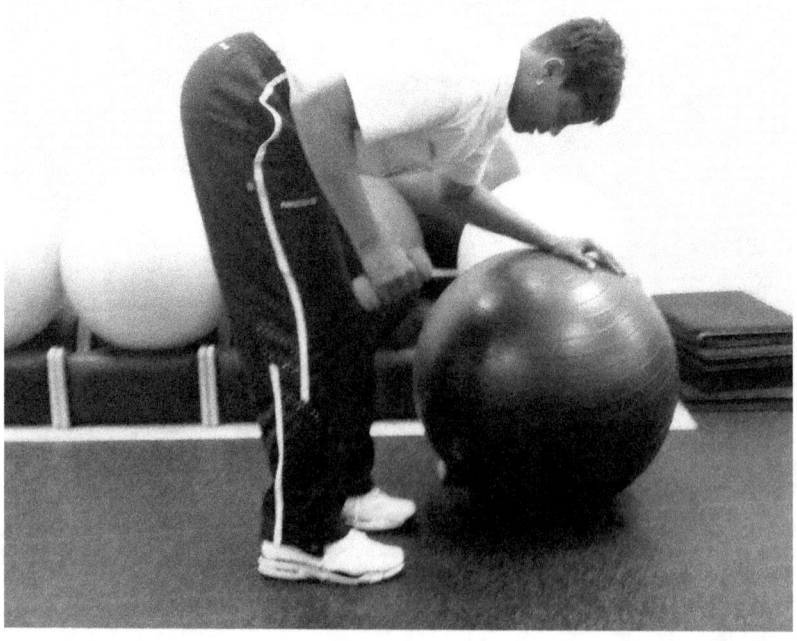

- Slowly extend your hand backwards.
- As you hand moves back, slowly turn your hand upward.

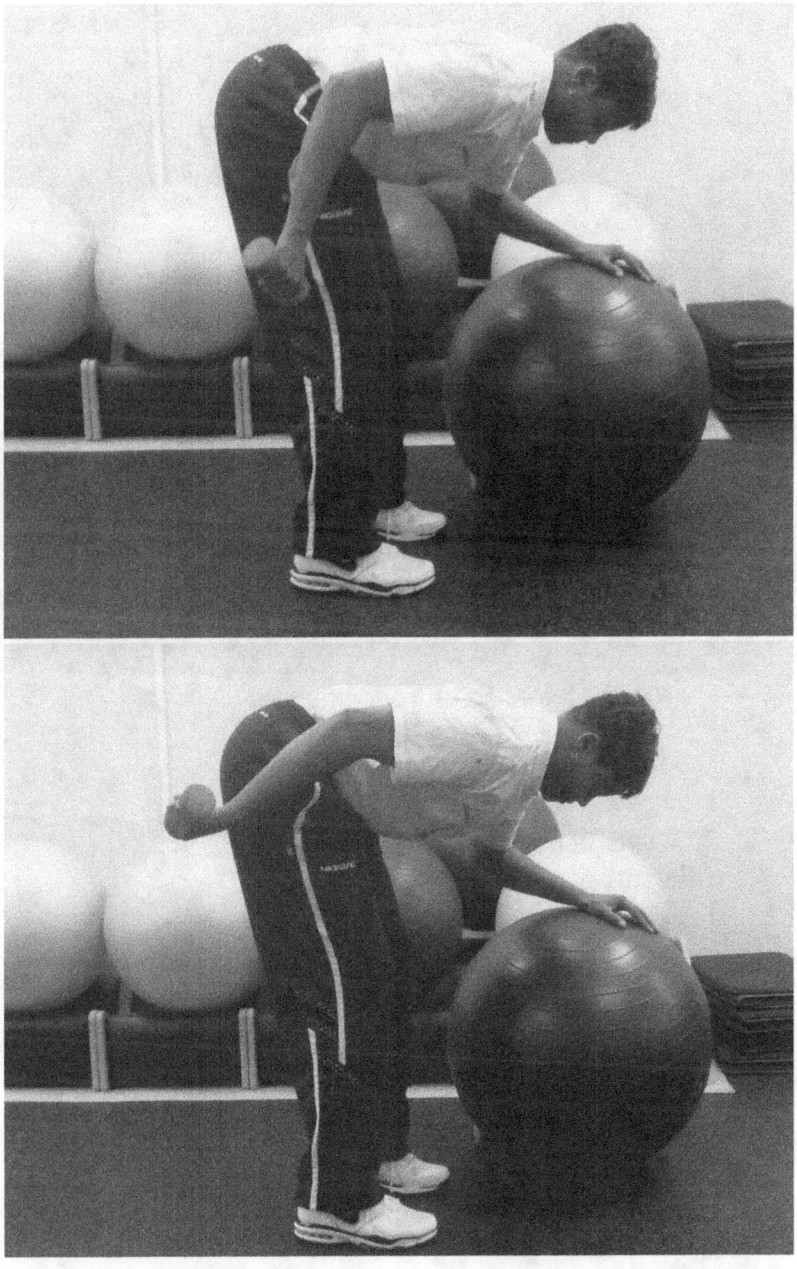

- The exercise is complete once your arm is fully extended, and your elbow is straight.

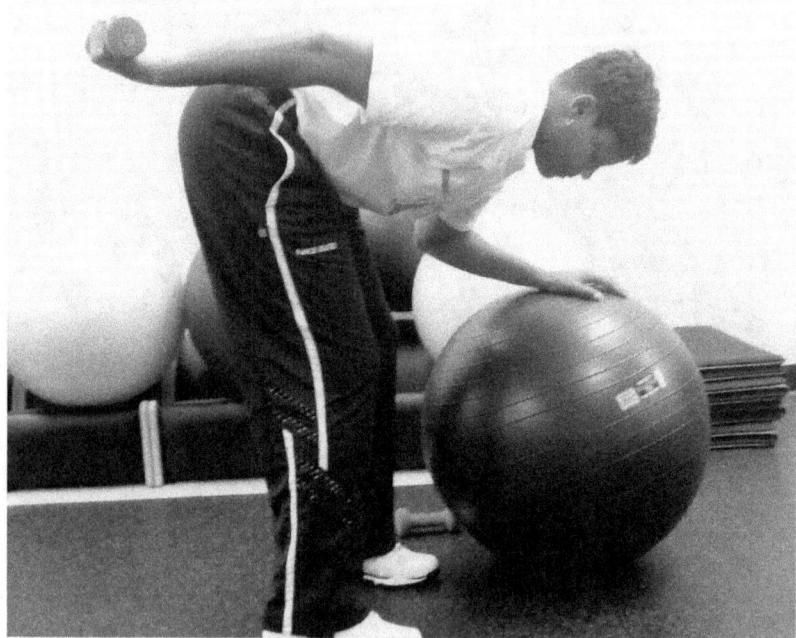

- Repeat exercise on your left side.

Progression as You Grow Stronger
1) 3 sets 6-8 repetitions
2) 3 sets of 8-10 repetitions
3) 3 sets of 10-12 repetitions

Leg Raise

- Press small of back into the floor.
- Keep abdominal muscles tight.
- Place hands at side for support.
- Keep foot flexed. Do not point toe.

Exercise Instructions

- Begin with both legs on the floor, back pressed into the floor.

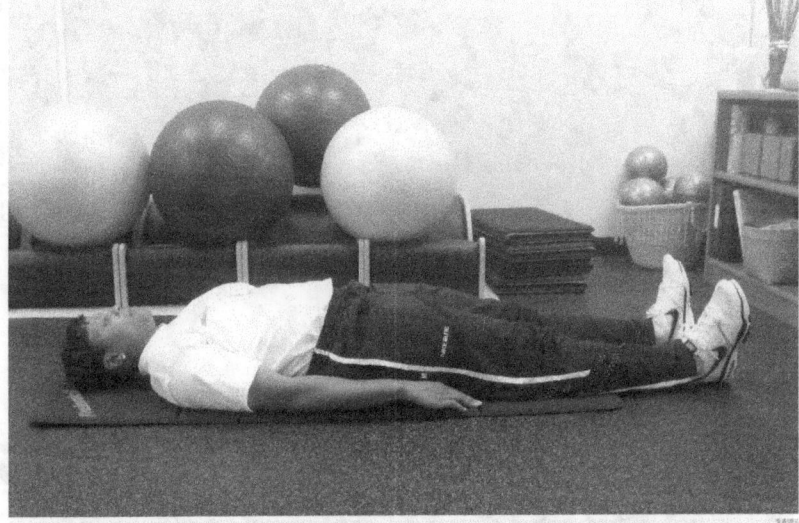

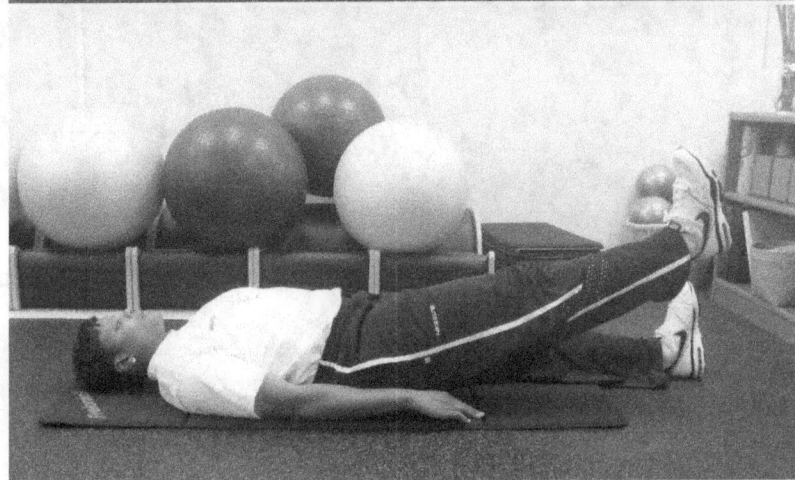

- Slowly lift right leg off the floor.

103

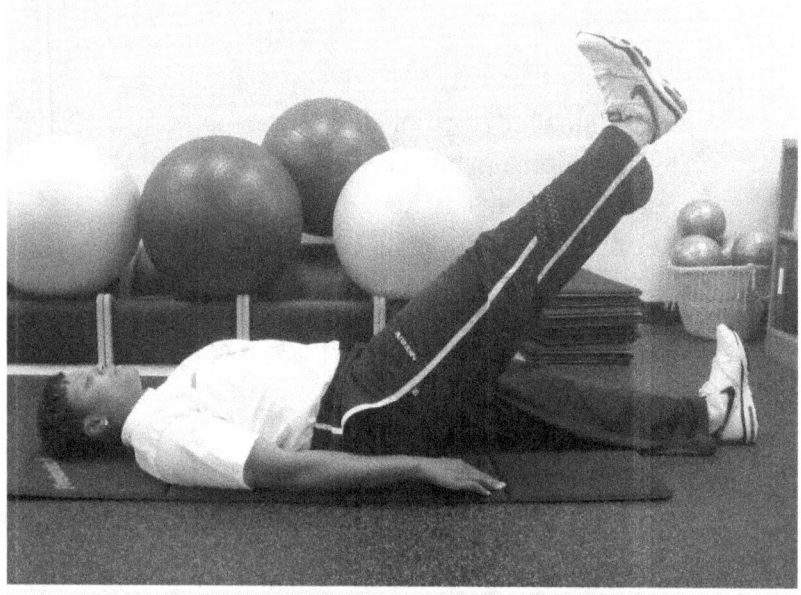

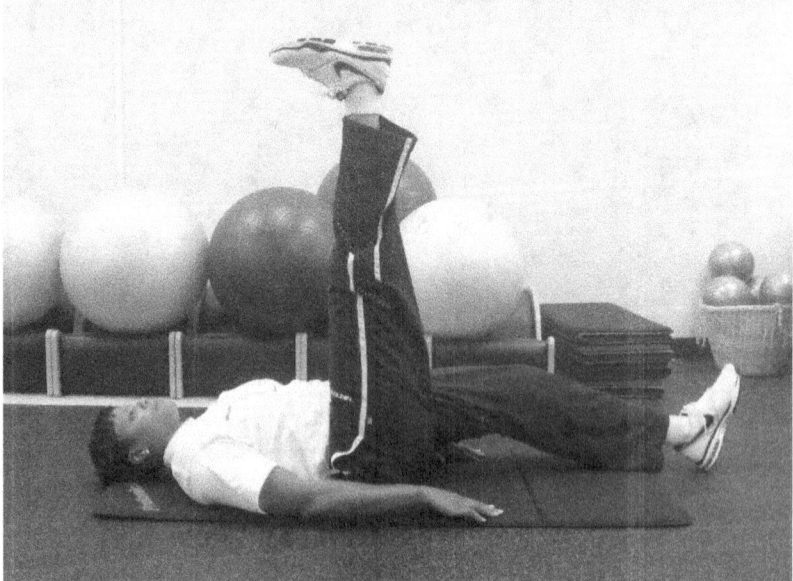

- Continue raising leg until the leg is at a right angle to the floor.
- Repeat with left leg.

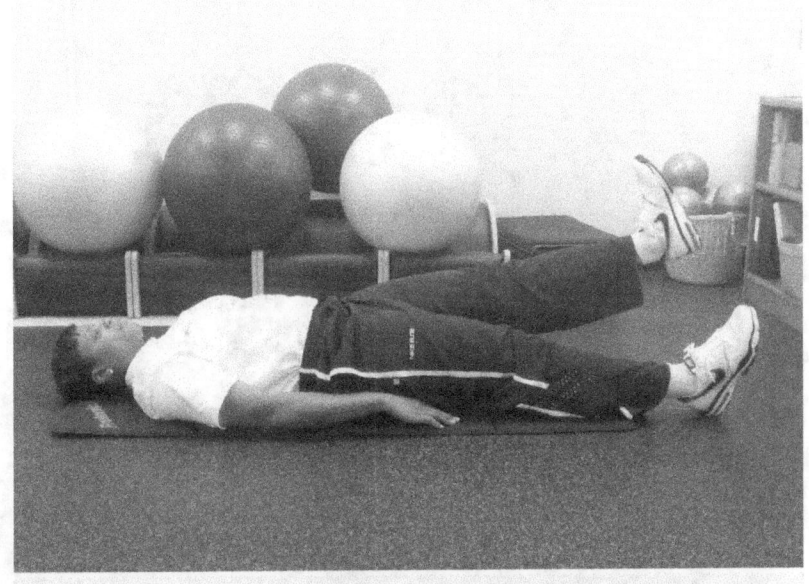

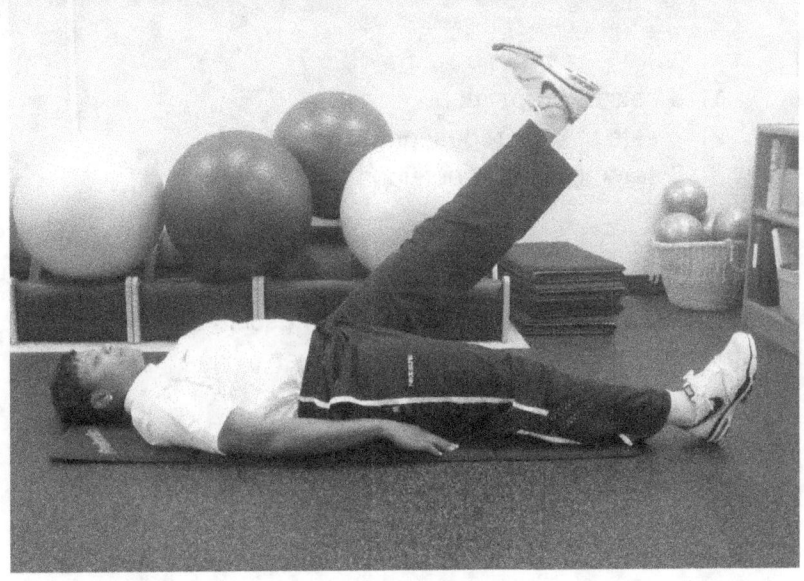

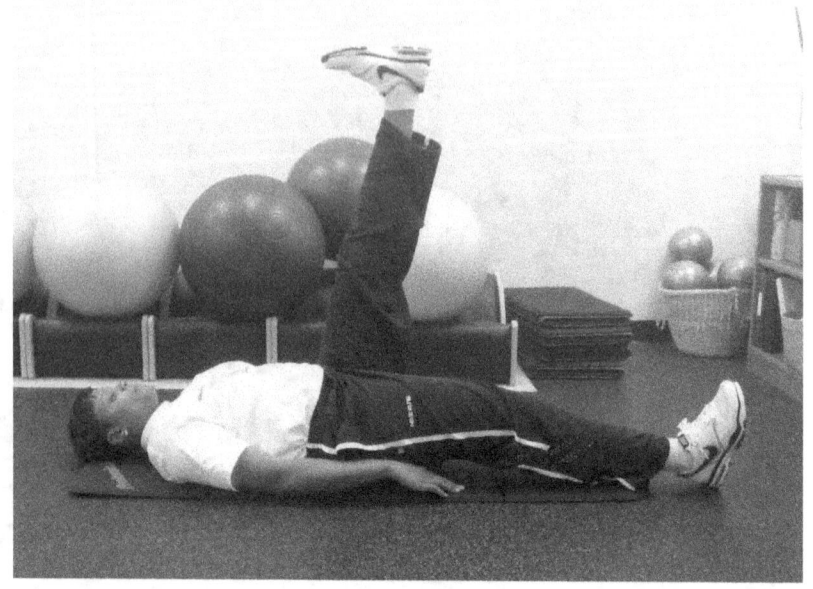

Progression as You Grow Stronger

1) 3 sets 6-8 repetitions
2) 3 sets of 8-10 repetitions
3) 3 sets of 10-12 repetitions

Note:

If you cannot raise your leg to a full 45 degree angle, raise it as high as you can. Your hamstring muscles will stretch over time and allow you to lift your leg higher.

Chair Squats

- Place a sturdy chair directly behind you.
- Keep your abdominal muscles tight throughout the exercise.
- Keep your knees behind your toes.

Exercise Instructions

- Stand about six inches in front of the chair.

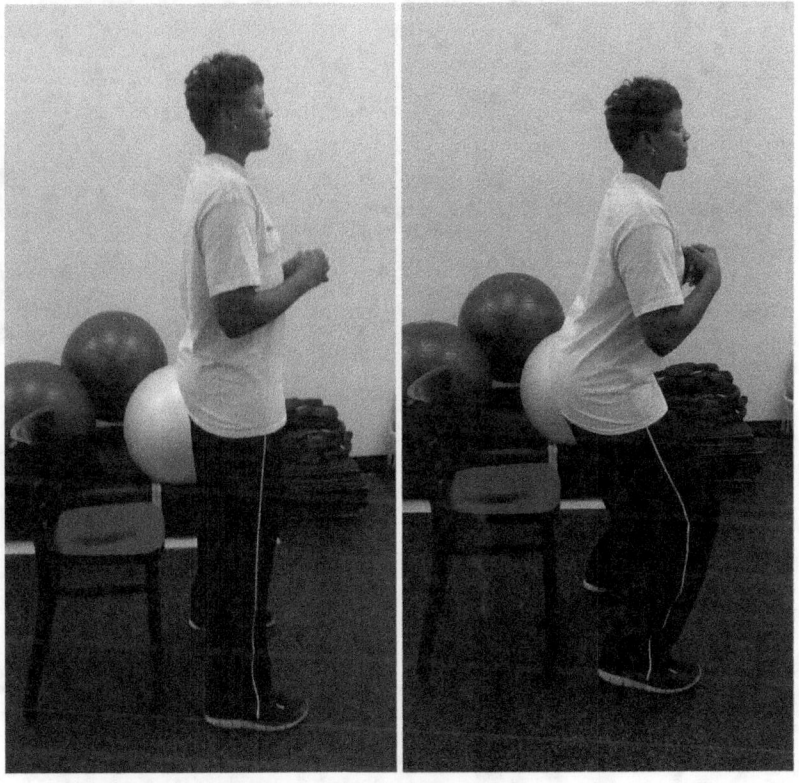

- Slowly lower yourself into the chair.

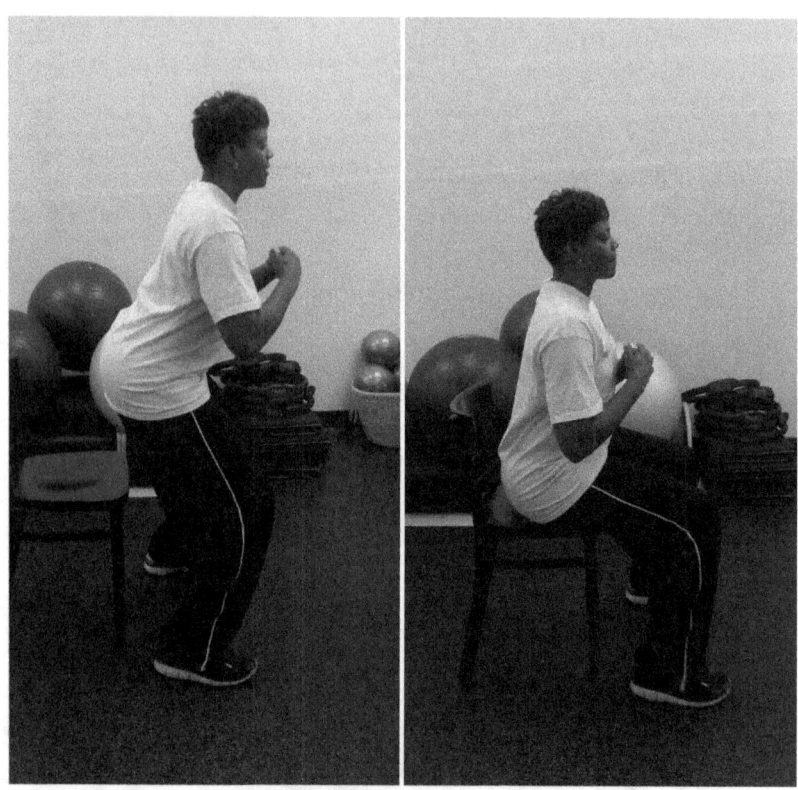

- Slowly return to a standing position.

Progression as You Grow Stronger
1) 3 sets 6-8 repetitions
2) 3 sets of 8-10 repetitions
3) 3 sets of 10-12 repetitions

Note:

As you grow more advanced, hover over the chair instead of making contact with the chair seat.

Hamstring Curl

Exercise Check List
- Use a sturdy chair.
- Keep your abdominal muscles tight throughout the exercise.
- Keep your knees slightly flexed to protect your knee joint from injury.
- Keep your foot flexed. Do not point your toes.

Exercise Instructions
- Place your hands on the back of the chair for balance.
- Lift your foot up toward your buttocks.

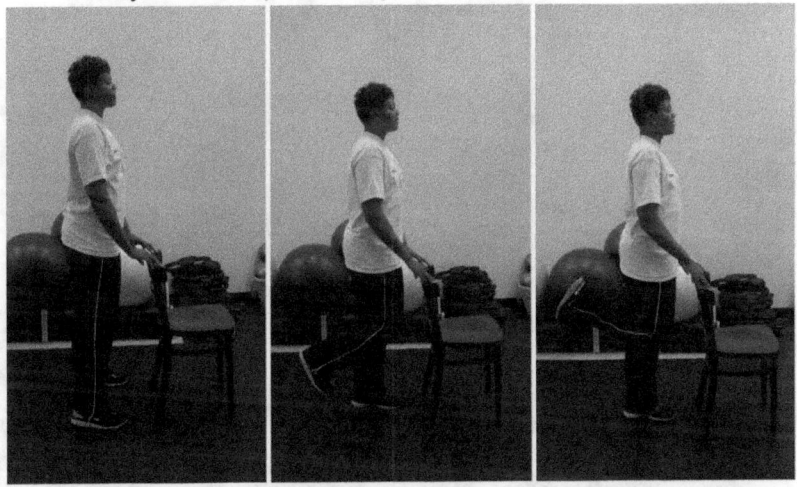

- Stop when your foot is just above your knee.
- Hold for a moment, then slowly lower foot toward the floor.
- Don't touch the floor with your foot until you have completed one set of repetitions on that side.
- Switch sides.

Progression as You Grow Stronger
1) 3 sets 6-8 repetitions
2) 3 sets of 8-10 repetitions
3) 3 sets of 10-12 repetitions

Calf Raises

Exercise Check List
- Use a sturdy chair.
- Keep your abdominal muscles tight throughout the exercise.
- Keep your knees slightly flexed to protect your knee joint from injury.

Exercise Instructions
- Place your hands on the back of the chair for balance.
- Lift your heels off the floor until your heels are as high as possible without going onto the tips of your toes.

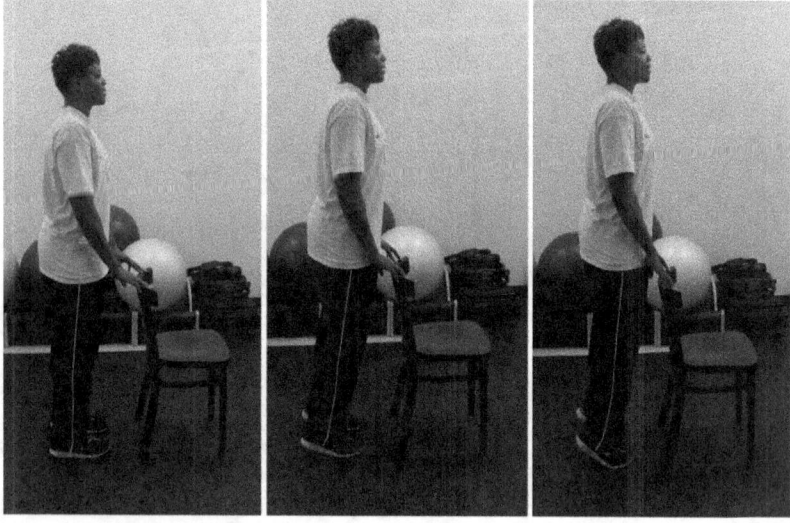

- Lower the heels back to the floor.

Progression as You Grow Stronger
1) 3 sets 6-8 repetitions
2) 3 sets of 8-10 repetitions
3) 3 sets of 10-12 repetitions

Note:
As you advance in strength, stand on a low step with just the ball and toes on the step. Start with heel lower than the step. This increases the stretch on the working muscles.

Abs on Physio Ball

Exercise Check List
- Keep your abdominal muscles tight throughout the exercise.
- Do not arch your back.

Exercise Instructions
- Position your knees and lower legs on the physio ball so your feet are on one side of the ball and your knees are on the other.

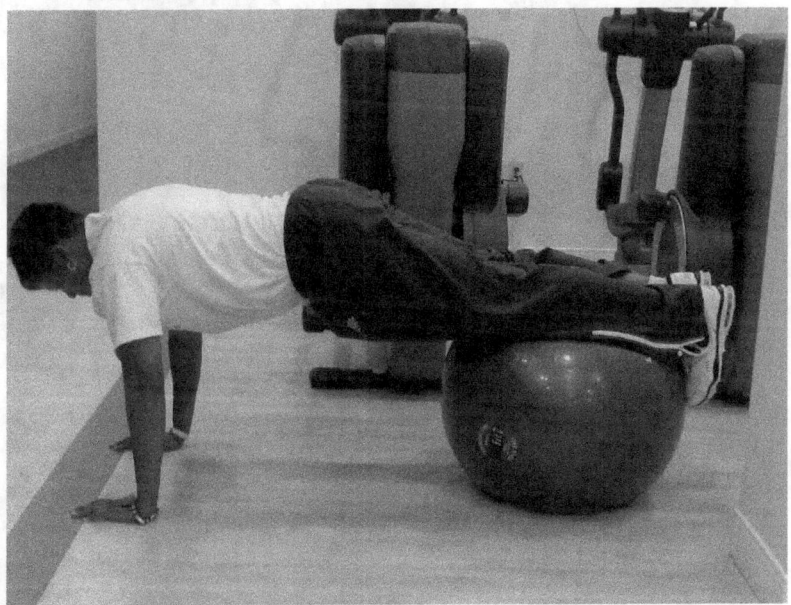

- Position your hands below your shoulders with your body straight.

111

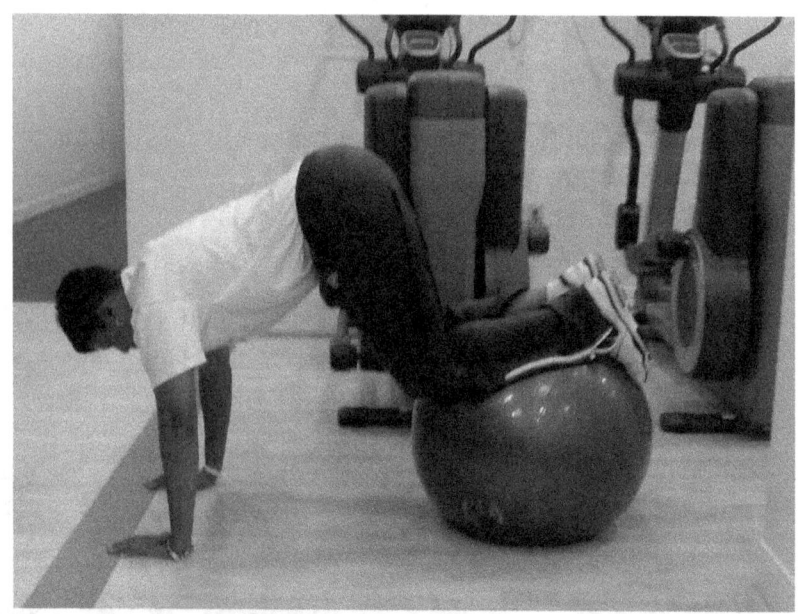

- Slowly bring the ball closer to your hands, allowing your buttocks to rise toward the ceiling.

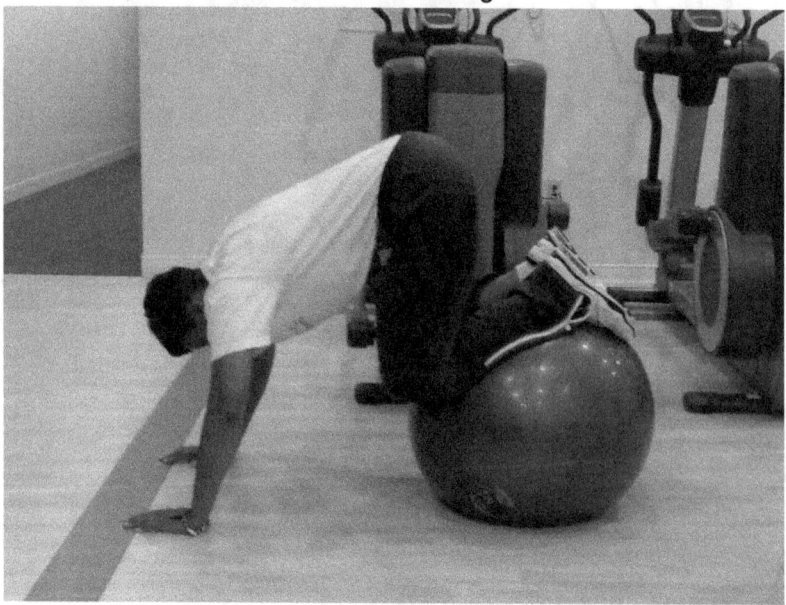

- When your ankles are at the top of the ball, and your knees begin to feel like they are going to slide off the ball, slowly reverse direction toward your starting position.

Progression as You Grow Stronger
1) 3 sets 6-8 repetitions
2) 3 sets of 8-10 repetitions
3) 3 sets of 10-12 repetitions

You may also perform pushups from the starting position for this exercise.

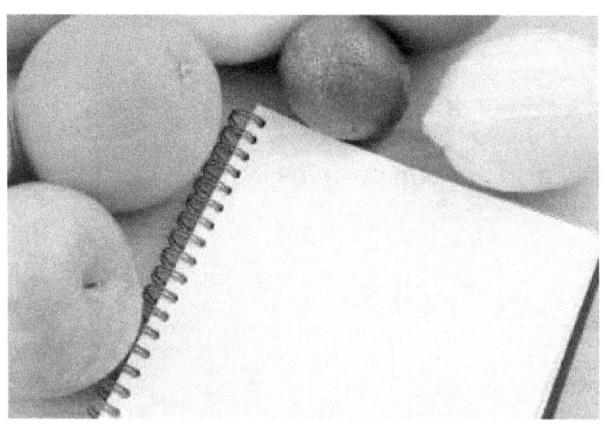

MEAL PLANNER

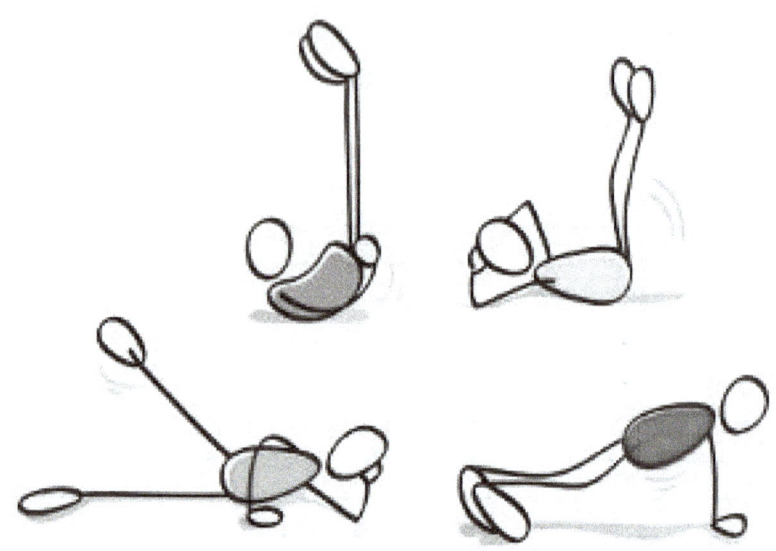

EXERCISE LOG

Increase your motivation. Log in your exercises!

Date_____ **Weight** _____

Day: Mon Tue Wed Thur Fri Sat Sun

Exercises	Sets	Repetitions	Weight
1._____			
2._____			
3._____			
4._____			
5._____			
6._____			
7._____			
8._____			

Date_____ **Weight** _____

Day: *Mon* *Tue* *Wed* *Thur* *Fri* *Sat* *Sun*

Exercises	Sets	Repetitions	Weight
1.			
2.			
3.			
4.			
5.			
6.			
7.			
8.			

Date_____ **Weight** _____

Day: *Mon* *Tue* *Wed* *Thur* *Fri* *Sat* *Sun*

Exercises	Sets	Repetitions	Weight
1.			
2.			
3.			
4.			
5.			
6.			
7.			
8.			

Date_____ Weight _____

Day: Mon Tue Wed Thur Fri Sat Sun

Exercises	Sets	Repetitions	Weight
1.			
2.			
3.			
4.			
5.			
6.			
7.			
8.			

Date_____ Weight _____

Day: Mon Tue Wed Thur Fri Sat Sun

Exercises	Sets	Repetitions	Weight
1.			
2.			
3.			
4.			
5.			
6.			
7.			
8.			

Date_____ Weight _____

Day: *Mon Tue Wed Thur Fri Sat Sun*

Exercises **Sets** **Repetitions** **Weight**

1._____

2._____

3._____

4._____

5._____

6._____

7._____

8._____

Date_____ Weight _____

Day: *Mon Tue Wed Thur Fri Sat Sun*

Exercises **Sets** **Repetitions** **Weight**

1._____

2._____

3._____

4._____

5._____

6._____

7._____

8._____

Date_____ Weight _____

Day: Mon Tue Wed Thur Fri Sat Sun

Exercises	Sets	Repetitions	Weight
1.			
2.			
3.			
4.			
5.			
6.			
7.			
8.			

Date_____ Weight _____

Day: Mon Tue Wed Thur Fri Sat Sun

Exercises	Sets	Repetitions	Weight
1.			
2.			
3.			
4.			
5.			
6.			
7.			
8.			

Date_____ Weight _____

Day: Mon Tue Wed Thur Fri Sat Sun

Exercises	**Sets**	**Repetitions**	**Weight**
1.			
2.			
3.			
4.			
5.			
6.			
7.			
8.			

Date_____ Weight _____

Day: Mon Tue Wed Thur Fri Sat Sun

Exercises	**Sets**	**Repetitions**	**Weight**
1.			
2.			
3.			
4.			
5.			
6.			
7.			
8.			

ABOUT THE AUTHOR

In February 2002, while playing professional basketball in Italy, Edna Campbell was elbowed in her breast. That opponent ended up being a blessing, because that blow quite possibly saved her life. That fateful day led to Edna discovering a mass in her right breast, and a subsequent breast cancer diagnosis. Edna would return to the states and miss most of her season with the WNBA's Sacramento Monarchs.

After having a lumpectomy, and receiving chemotherapy, Edna was determined to get back on the basketball court. While still undergoing radiation, she took to the court. A crowd on their feet, overcome with emotion, applauded Edna's entry into the game. WNBA fans recalled and voted August 13, 2002 one of the most inspirational moments in the history of the Women's National Basketball Association—the day Edna Campbell sported a bald head, and entered the game.

Inspired by her experience, Edna's passion is to make a difference in the lives of those who are going through a diagnosis, and to educate them on how to fully recover from the treatment. Edna's approach to her recovery not only allowed her to regain the stamina and strength to compete as a professional athlete, but it enables her to live a vibrant, healthy life rooted in healthy lifestyle choices.

Edna Campbell resides in California. Her life is dedicated to empowering, and educating survivors to be a shining example of strength and assuming personal responsibility for their health. Through her recovery system Edna strives to make a tangible difference in lives.

Edna Campbell can also be booked to share her riveting, eye-opening, incredibly inspiring story. Contact her through http://ednacampbell.com.